Table of contents

Delicious Apple Granola Breakfast	
Mango Oats	
Delicious Banana and Coconut Oatmeal	5
Fruity Bowls	5
Carrot and Zucchini Oatmeal	5
Wild Rice Bowls	6
Coconut Quinoa Mix	6
Maple Apricots and Rice Mix	6
Simple Banana Bread	6
Cinnamon Apple Bowls	6
Greek Dash Casserole	6
Easy Breakfast Casserole	7
Blueberries Oatmeal	7
Mexican Dash Diet Eggs	7
Tomato Pomegranate Bowls	7
Simple Apple Oatmeal	8
Banana, Rice and Chia Bowls	8
Quinoa And Oats	8
Radish and Eggs Mix	8
Pumpkin Oatmeal	8
Raspberry Oatmeal	9
Peppers Eggs Mix	9
Delicious Frittata	9
Spinach Frittata	9
Potato and Shrimp Bowls	9
Breakfast Veggie Omelet	10
Scrambled Eggs	10
Cilantro Hash	10
Apple And Raisins Oatmeal	10
Delicious Peanut Butter Oats	10
Black Beans and Eggs Salad	11
Orange And Strawberry Breakfast Mix	11
Omelet	11
Orange Hash Mix	11
Fruits and Cereals Mix	12
Breakfast Berries Compote	12
Shrimp and Eggs	12
Apples and Dates Oatmeal	12
Sweet Rice Bowls	12
Scrambled Eggs and Veggies	13
Mexican Casserole	13
Quinoa and Tomato Bowls	13
Shrimp Frittata	13

Raisin Rice Bowls	14
Corn Pudding	14
Sweet Potatoes Mix	15
Shrimp Salad	15
Almond and Cherries Oats	15
Cranberry Toast	15
Strawberry and Chia Bowls	15
Burrito Bowls	16
Spiced Coconut Oats	16
Apples and Apricots Bowls	16
Carrot Oatmeal	16
Blueberries Oatmeal	17
Orange and Avocado Quinoa	17
Tofu and Veggies Frittata	17
Coconut Hash Bowls	17
Chia Pudding	17
Breakfast Potatoes	18
Nutmeg Oatmeal	18
Breakfast Nuts and Squash Bowls	18
Leeks, Kale and Sweet Potato Mix	18
Brown Rice and Plums	18
Egg Casserole	19
Maple Apples	19
Quinoa and Eggs Mix	19
Apples and Sauce	19
Sweet Potato and Sausage Pie	20
Eggs and Bacon Mix	20
Pumpkin Butter	20
Pineapple and Carrot Mix	20
Ginger and Spring Onions Eggs Mix	20
Spinach Pie	21
Creamy Veggie Omelet	21
Sausage and Hash Browns	21
Salmon Omelet	21
Chicken Omelet	22
Chicken Tacos	22
Coconut Turkey Mix	22
Quinoa Casserole	22
Quinoa Curry	23
Shrimp and Green Beans Mix	23
Delicious Black Bean Chili	23

Chicken Stew	23	Lemon and Spinach Trout	34
Chicken and Veggies	24	Lentils and Shrimp Soup	34
Succulent Beef Roast	24	Mexican Chicken	34
Chicken and Peppers Soup	24	Oregano Turkey Mix	35
Turkey Chili	24	Chicken Breast Stew	35
Creamy Beef Mix	25	Turkey Breast and Sweet Potato Mix	35
Pulled Chicken	25	Creamy Pork Chops	36
Lime Chicken Mix	25	Italian Chicken	36
Mediterranean Chicken	25	Chicken Breast and Cinnamon Veggie Mix	36
Chicken and Mushroom Soup	26	Paprika Pork and Broccoli	36
Delicious Veggie Soup	26	Mexican Beef Mix	36
Turkey and Tomatoes	26	Maple Beef Tenderloin	37
Chicken and Rice Soup	26	Mushroom Cream	37
Delicious Black Bean Soup	27	Beef and Cabbage Stew	37
Ginger Beef Mix	27	Greek Beef	37
Beet Soup	27	Garlic Chicken Mix	38
Tarragon Chicken and Corn	27	Roast and Veggies	38
Delicious Tomato Cream	28	Beef Roast Soup	38
Shrimp and Rice	28	Cod Soup	38
Rich Lentils Soup	28	Coconut Salmon Soup	39
Broccoli and Cauliflower Soup	28	Ground Beef and Veggies Soup	39
Pork Chops and Sprouts	29	Shrimp and Asparagus	39
Butternut Squash Cream	29	Greek Cod Mix	39
Chickpeas Mix	29	Creamy Fish Curry	39
Red Beans and Chicken Mix	29	Hot Mackerel	40
Navy Beans Stew	30	Lemon and Basil Sea Bass	40
Potatoes Stew	30	Mussels Mix	40
Broccoli Soup	30	Turkey Wings and Veggies	40
Easy Navy Beans Soup	30	Pork Chops and Cabbage	41
Turkey Soup	30	Citrus Turkey Mix	41
Black Beans and Mango Mix	31	Zucchini and Sprouts Salad	41
Spinach Soup	31	Broccoli Mix	41
Shrimp and Quinoa Mix	31	Tasty Bean Side Dish	41
Asian Salmon	31	Green Beans	42
Seafood Stew	32	Creamy Corn	42
Chicken and Potatoes	32	Classic Peas and Carrots	42
Slow Cooked Tuna	32	Mushroom Pilaf	42
Herbed Salmon	32	Lime Fennel	43
Green Beans Soup	33	Butternut Mix	43
Coconut Clams	33	Sausage Side Dish	43
Beef and Carrots	33	Easy Potatoes Mix	43
Creamy Seafood and Veggies Soup	33	Black-Eyed Peas Mix	43
Beef Chili Mix	34	Green Beans and Corn Mix	44
Seafood Gumbo	34	Minty Brussels Sprouts	44

Spiced Carrots	44
Squash and Grains Mix	44
Mushroom Mix	45
Spinach and Rice	45
Green Beans Salad	45
Creamy Mushrooms Mix	45
Ginger Beets	45
Artichokes Mix	46
Creamy Corn	46
Asparagus Mix	46
Black Bean and Corn Mix	46
Celery Mix	46
Kale Side Dish	47
Spicy Eggplant	47
Corn Salad	47
Spinach and Sprouts Salad	47
Spiced Cabbage	48
Spinach and Beans Mix	48
Sage Sweet Potatoes	48
Garlicky Potato Mash	48
Creamy Cauliflower	48
Chickpeas Side Dish	49
Warm Eggplant Salad	49
Garlic and Rosemary Potato Mix	49
Apple Brussels sprouts	49
Tomato Salad	50
Italian Beans Mix	50
Tomatoes, Okra and Zucchini Mix	50
Easy Cabbage	50
Acorn Squash Mix	50
Spring Onions and Peas Mix	51
Italian Zucchini and Squash	51
Coconut Broccoli	51
Asian Green Beans	51
Cauliflower Rice and Mushrooms	51
Cranberries, Cauliflower and Mushroom Mix	52
Creamy Cauliflower Rice	52
Curry Zucchini Mix	52
Creamy and Cheesy Spinach	52
Dill Cauliflower Mash	52
Baby Spinach and Avocado Mix	53
Simple Parsnips Mix	53
Basil and Oregano Mushrooms	53
Minty Okra	53
Cabbage, Radish and Carrot Mix	53
Simple Swiss Chard Mix	54
Eggplant Salsa	54
Zucchini Dip	54
Artichoke and Beans Spread	54
Stuffed White Mushrooms	55
Italian Tomato Appetizer	55
Cauliflower Dip	55
Sweet Pineapple Snack	55
Chickpeas Hummus	55
Asparagus Snack	56
Shrimp and Beans Appetizer Salad	56
Mushroom Salsa	56
Pepper and Chickpeas Dip	56
White Bean Spread	57
Minty Spinach Dip	57
Turnips and Cauliflower Spread	57
Shrimp and Zucchini Salad	57
Italian Veggie Dip	57
Cajun Peas Spread	58
Cashew Spread	58
Coconut Spinach Dip	58
Black Bean Salsa	58
Mango and Olives Salsa	58
Chili Coconut Corn Spread	59
Artichoke and Spinach Dip	59
Mushroom and Bell Pepper Dip	59
Warm French Veggie Salad	59
Bulgur and Beans Salad	60
Salmon Salad	60
Pineapple Chicken Wings	60
Spiced Pecans Snack	60
Beef Party Meatballs	61
Beef Rolls	61
Shrimp Dip	61
Tomato Salsa	61
White Fish Sticks	61
Tomato Shrimp Salad	62
Green Beans Salsa	62
Stuffed Chicken	62
Italian Nuts Mix	62
Dill Walnuts and Seeds Mix	63
Kale Dip	63
Tomato Dip	63

Zucchini Dip	63
Easy Zucchini Rolls	63
Jumbo Shrimp Appetizer	64
Black Beans Salsa	64
Salmon Appetizer Salad	64
Beet and Celery Spread	64
Clams Salad	64
Creamy Endive Salad	65
Chili Cauliflower Dip	65
Cranberries, Apple and Onion Salad	65
Sausage Meatballs and Apricot Sauce	65
Sriracha Chicken Dip	66
Shrimp Cocktail	66
Cod Salsa	66
Salmon and Carrots Appetizer Salad	66
Italian Shrimp Salad	66
Salmon and Scallions Salad	67
Salmon Bites and Lemon Dressing	67
Easy Carrot and Pineapple Cake	67
Mango Cake	67
Coconut Green Tea Cream	67
Sweet Coconut Figs	68
Avocado and Cashews Cake	68
Chocolate and Vanilla Cream	68
Cinnamon Tomato Mix	68
Tomato Pie	68
Mint Cream	69
Berries and Orange Sauce	69
Mango and Orange Sauce	69
Sweet Minty Grapefruit Mix	69
Coconut Banana Cream	69
Plums Stew	70
Cinnamon Apples	70
Figs and Avocado Bowls	70
Cocoa Cake	70
Blueberry Pie	70
Coconut Peach Cobbler	71
Cherry and Chocolate Cream	71
Poached Strawberries	71
Poached Bananas	71
Orange and Pecans Cake	71
Plums Cake	72
Poached Pears	72
Pumpkin Pie	72
Carrot Muffins	72
Lemon Cream	72
Minty Rhubarb Dip	73
Cherry Jam	73
Cinnamon Rice Pudding	73
Orange and Plums Compote	73
Almond Chocolate Bars	73
Pineapple Pudding	74
Delicious Apple Mix	74
Grapes Compote	74
Avocado Pudding	74
Chia Pudding	74
Grapefruit Compote	74
Dark Cherry and Cocoa Compote	75
Creamy Grapes Bowls	75
Citrus Apples and Pears Mix	75
Pears Cake	75
Walnuts and Avocado Bowls	75
Cocoa Pudding	76
Raspberry Energy Bars	76
Berries Cream	76
Apple and Rice Bowls	76
Blackberries and Cocoa Pudding	76
Peach Compote	76
Zucchini Cake	77
Maple Apple Bowls	77
Grapes Pudding	77
Apricot Cream	77
Poached Apples	77
Lemon Cream	78
Stewed Cardamom Pears	78
Maple Grapes Compote	78
Brown Rice Pudding	78
Berries Compote	78
Berry Cobbler	78
Pumpkin Apple Dip	79
Vanilla Apple, Plums and Grapes Bowls	79
Apple Dip	79
Sweet Pumpkin and Avocado Cream	79
Cranberry Dip	79
Apple Cake	80
Sweet Mango Dip	80
Plum Dip	80
Plum and Berries Bowls	80

Dash Diet Slow Cooker Breakfast Recipes

Delicious Apple Granola Breakfast

Preparation time: 10 minutes | Cooking time: 0 minutes | Servings: 4

Ingredients:

- 2 green apples, peeled, cored and cut into medium chunks
- 1 teaspoon cinnamon powder
- ½ cup granola
- ½ cup bran flakes
- 2 tablespoons dairy free butter
- ½ teaspoon nutmeg, ground
- ¼ cup natural apple juice
- 1 teaspoon stevia

Directions:

1. In your slow cooker, mix the apples with the granola, bran flakes, apple juice, stevia, butter, nutmeg and cinnamon, toss, cover and cook on Low for 4 hours.
2. Divide into bowls and serve.

Nutrition: Calories 129, Fat .8.1g, Cholesterol 0mg, Sodium 50mg, Carbohydrate 39.6g, Fiber 6.8g, Sugars 21.5g, Protein 5.5g, Potassium 331mg

Mango Oats

Preparation time: 10 minutes | Cooking time: 3 hours | Servings: 4

Ingredients:

- 1 mango, peeled and cubed
- 2 cups non-fat milk
- 1 cup old-fashioned oats
- ½ teaspoon almond extract
- ½ tablespoon sugar

Directions:

1. In your slow cooker, combine the oats with the milk and the other ingredients, toss, put the lid on and cook on High for 3 hours.
2. Divide into bowls into bowls and serve for breakfast.

Nutrition: Calories 178, Fat .1.6g, Cholesterol 2mg, Sodium 67mg, Carbohydrate 33.7g, Fiber 3.3g, Sugars 19.2g, Protein 7.3g, Potassium 404mg

Delicious Banana and Coconut Oatmeal

Preparation time: 10 minutes | Cooking time: 7 hours | Servings: 4

Ingredients:

- 2 cups banana, peeled and sliced
- 28 ounces coconut milk
- ½ cup water
- ½ teaspoon vanilla extract
- 1 tablespoon flax seed
- 1 tablespoon dairy free butter
- ¼ teaspoon nutmeg, ground
- ½ teaspoon cinnamon powder
- 1 cup old-fashioned rolled oats
- 2 tablespoons stevia

Directions:

1. In your slow cooker, combine the banana with the milk, water, oats, stevia, butter, nutmeg, cinnamon, vanilla and flax seed, toss a bit, cover and cook on Low for 7 hours.
2. Divide into bowls and serve.

Nutrition: Calories 614, Fat .49.7g, Cholesterol 0mg, Sodium 35mg, Carbohydrate 43g, Fiber 8.9g, Sugars 16.5g, Protein 8.4g, Potassium 879mg

Fruity Bowls

Preparation time: 10 minutes | Cooking time: 1 hour | Servings: 4

Ingredients:

- 1 cup apple, peeled, cored and cubed
- 1 cup blackberries
- 2 cups non-fat milk
- 2 tablespoons sugar
- ½ cup pears, peeled, cored and cubed
- ½ teaspoon vanilla extract

Directions:

1. In your slow cooker, combine the fruits with the milk and the other ingredients, put the lid on and cook on High for 1 hour.
2. Divide the mix into bowls and serve.

Nutrition: Calories 125, Fat .0.3g, Cholesterol 2mg, Sodium 66mg, Carbohydrate 26.3g, Fiber 3.9g, Sugars 21.6g, Protein 4.7g, Potassium 332mg

Carrot and Zucchini Oatmeal

Preparation time: 10 minutes | Cooking time: 8 hours | Servings: 4

Ingredients:

- ½ cup gluten-free oats
- 1 carrot, grated
- ¼ teaspoon cloves, ground
- ¼ cup walnuts, chopped
- ½ teaspoon cinnamon powder
- 1 and ½ cups coconut milk
- ¼ zucchini, grated
- ¼ teaspoon nutmeg, ground
- 2 tablespoons stevia

Directions:

1. In your slow cooker, combine the oats with the carrot, zucchini, milk, nutmeg, cloves, cinnamon and stevia, cover and cook on Low for 8 hours.
2. Divide into bowls, sprinkle walnuts on top and serve.

Nutrition: Calories 321, Fat .27.3g, Cholesterol 0mg, Sodium 26mg, Carbohydrate 25.5g, Fiber 5.3g, Sugars 4.1g, Protein 6.1g, Potassium 360mg

Wild Rice Bowls

Preparation time: 10 minutes | Cooking time: 2 hours | Servings: 4

Ingredients:
- 1 cup wild rice
- ½ cup spring onions, chopped
- ½ cup cherry tomatoes, halved
- 2 cups water
- 1 teaspoon rosemary, dried
- A pinch of salt and black pepper

Directions:
1. In your slow cooker, combine the rice with the water and the other ingredients, put the lid on and cook on High for 2 hours.
2. Stir the mix more time, divide it into bowls and serve for breakfast.

Nutrition: Calories 152, Fat .0.6g, Cholesterol 0mg, Sodium 10mg, Carbohydrate 32g, Fiber 3.2g, Sugars 1.9g, Protein 6.3g, Potassium 263mg

Coconut Quinoa Mix

Preparation time: 10 minutes | Cooking time: 4 hours | Servings: 4

Ingredients:
- 1 teaspoon vanilla extract
- 1 cup quinoa
- 1/8 coconut flakes
- ¼ cup cranberries
- 2 teaspoons stevia
- 3 cups coconut water
- 1/8 cup almonds, sliced

Directions:
1. In your slow cooker, mix the coconut water with the quinoa, vanilla, stevia, coconut, almonds and cranberries, cover and cook on Low for 4 hours.
2. Stir the quinoa mix, divide it between plates and serve for breakfast.

Nutrition: Calories 259, Fat .8.6g, Cholesterol 0mg, Sodium 194mg, Carbohydrate 39.3g, Fiber 6.7g, Sugars 6g, Protein 8.4g, Potassium 768mg

Maple Apricots and Rice Mix

Preparation time: 10 minutes | Cooking time: 3 hours | Servings: 4

Ingredients:
- 2 cups non-fat milk
- 1 cup wild rice
- 2 tablespoons maple syrup
- ½ teaspoon vanilla extract
- ½ cup apricots, chopped
- ¼ teaspoon cinnamon powder

Directions:
1. In your slow cooker, combine the rice with the milk and the other ingredients, toss, put the lid on and cook on High for 3 hours.
2. Divide into bowls and serve for breakfast.

Nutrition: Calories 225, Fat .0.6g, Cholesterol 2mg, Sodium 69mg, Carbohydrate 44.9g, Fiber 2.9g, Sugars 14.8g, Protein 10.1g, Potassium 432mg

Simple Banana Bread

Preparation time: 10 minutes | Cooking time: 4 hours | Servings: 4

Ingredients:
- 2 eggs
- ½ teaspoon baking soda
- 3 bananas, peeled and mashed
- 2 cups whole wheat flour
- 1 teaspoon baking powder
- 2 tablespoons olive oil

Directions:
1. In a bowl, mix the eggs with the oil, flour, baking powder and baking soda and whisk well.
2. Add bananas, stir the batter, pour it into your greased slow cooker, cover and cook on Low for 4 hours.
3. Slice the bread, divide it between plates and serve.

Nutrition: Calories 399, Fat .10.1g, Cholesterol 82mg, Sodium 193mg, Carbohydrate 68.7g, Fiber 4g, Sugars 11.2g, Protein 10.2g, Potassium 539mg

Cinnamon Apple Bowls

Preparation time: 10 minutes | Cooking time: 2 hours | Servings: 4

Ingredients:
- 1 cup apples, cored and cut into wedges
- 1 cup low-fat milk
- 2 teaspoons cinnamon powder
- 2 teaspoons sugar

Directions:
1. In your slow cooker, combine the apples with the sugar and the other ingredients, put the lid on and cook on High for 2 hours.
2. Divide into bowls and serve.

Nutrition: Calories 62, Fat .0.7g, Cholesterol 3mg, Sodium 27mg, Carbohydrate 12.7g, Fiber 1.4g, Sugars 11g, Protein 2.2g, Potassium 151mg

Greek Dash Casserole

Preparation time: 10 minutes | Cooking time: 4 hours | Servings: 6

Ingredients:
- Black pepper to the taste
- 12 eggs, whisked
- 1 cup baby bell mushrooms, sliced
- 2 cups spinach
- ½ cup low-fat milk
- 1 tablespoon red onion, chopped
- 1 teaspoon garlic, minced

Directions:
1. In a bowl, mix the eggs with black pepper, milk, onion, garlic, mushrooms and spinach, toss, pour into your slow cooker, cover and cook on Low for 4 hours.
2. Slice, divide between plates and serve.

Nutrition: Calories 162, Fat .10g, Cholesterol 328mg, Sodium 328mg, Carbohydrate 5.6g, Fiber 0.5g, Sugars 3.6g, Protein 12.6g, Potassium 246mg

Easy Breakfast Casserole

Preparation time: 10 minutes | Cooking time: 4 hours | Servings: 8

Ingredients:
- A pinch of black pepper
- 8 eggs
- 1 teaspoon garlic, minced
- ½ yellow onion, chopped
- 2 bell peppers, chopped
- ¾ cup low-fat milk
- 2 teaspoons mustard
- 1 small broccoli head, florets separated
- 30 ounces hash browns

Directions:
1. In a bowl, mix the eggs with the milk, mustard, garlic, hash browns, onion, bell peppers, broccoli and black pepper, stir, pour into your slow cooker, cover and cook on Low for 4 hours.
2. Divide between plates and serve.

Nutrition: Calories 373, Fat .18.3g, Cholesterol 165mg, Sodium 438mg, Carbohydrate 42.5g, Fiber 4.2g, Sugars 5.1g, Protein 10.3g, Potassium 796mg

Blueberries Oatmeal

Preparation time: 10 minutes | Cooking time: 2 hours | Servings: 4

Ingredients:
- 2 cups non-fat milk
- 1 cup old fashioned oats
- 1 cup blueberries
- 2 teaspoons sugar
- ½ teaspoon cinnamon powder
- ½ teaspoon vanilla extract
- ½ teaspoon almond extract

Directions:
1. In your slow cooker, combine the oats with the milk, berries and the other ingredients, put the lid on and cook on High for 2 hours.
2. Divide the oatmeal into bowls and serve for breakfast.

Nutrition: Calories 231, Fat .2.7g, Cholesterol 2mg, Sodium 65mg, Carbohydrate 40.2g, Fiber 4.8g, Sugars 12.7g, Protein 9.3g, Potassium 391mg

Mexican Dash Diet Eggs

Preparation time: 5 minutes | Cooking time: 2 hours | Servings: 8

Ingredients:
- 12 ounces low-fat cheese, shredded
- 1 garlic clove, minced
- 1 cup nonfat sour cream
- 10 eggs
- Olive oil cooking spray
- 5 ounces canned green chilies, drained
- 10 ounces tomato sauce, sodium-free
- ½ teaspoon chili powder
- Black pepper to the taste

Directions:
1. In a bowl, mix the eggs with the cheese, sour cream, chili powder, black pepper, garlic, green chilies and tomato sauce, whisk, pour into your slow cooker after you've greased it with cooking oil, cover and cook on Low for 2 hours.
2. Divide between plates and serve.

Nutrition: Calories 395, Fat .27.5g, Cholesterol 262mg, Sodium 700mg, Carbohydrate 18.8g, Fiber 5.8g, Sugars 10.6g, Protein 20.9g, Potassium 610mg

Tomato Pomegranate Bowls

Preparation time: 10 minutes | Cooking time: 1 hour | Servings: 4

Ingredients:
- 1 cup pomegranate seeds
- ½ cup low-sodium veggie stock
- ½ pound cherry tomatoes, halved
- 1 teaspoon turmeric powder
- 1 tablespoon basil, chopped
- A pinch of cayenne pepper

Directions:
1. In your slow cooker, combine the tomatoes with the pomegranate seeds and the other ingredients, put the lid on and cook on High for 1 hour.
2. Divide into bowls and serve.

Nutrition: Calories 57, Fat .0.2g, Cholesterol 0mg, Sodium 21mg, Carbohydrate 13.2g, Fiber 1.3g, Sugars 6.8g, Protein 1g, Potassium 151mg

Simple Apple Oatmeal

Preparation time: 5 minutes | Cooking time: 10 hours | Servings: 4

Ingredients:
- 2 teaspoons low-fat butter
- 4 apples, peeled, cored and chopped
- 1 and ½ tablespoon cinnamon powder
- 1 cup coconut sugar
- 2 cups old-fashioned oats
- 4 cups coconut water

Directions:
1. Grease your slow cooker with the butter, add apples, coconut sugar, cinnamon, oats and water, cover and cook on Low for 10 hours.
2. Stir the oatmeal, divide into bowls and serve.

Nutrition: Calories 421, Fat .30g, Cholesterol 0mg, Sodium 40mg, Carbohydrate 43g, Fiber 8.2g, Sugars 27.4g, Protein 4.1g, Potassium 554mg

Banana, Rice and Chia Bowls

Preparation time: 10 minutes | Cooking time: 2 hours | Servings: 4

Ingredients:
- 2 cups non-fat milk
- 1 cup brown rice
- 2 bananas, peeled and sliced
- 1 tablespoon maple syrup
- 2 tablespoons chia seeds
- 1 teaspoon sugar
- 1 teaspoon vanilla extract
- 1 teaspoon cinnamon powder

Directions:
1. In your slow cooker, combine the milk with the bananas, maple syrup and the other ingredients, put the lid on and cook on High for 2 hours.
2. Divide the mix into bowls and serve for breakfast.

Nutrition: Calories 321, Fat .3.5g, Cholesterol 3mg, Sodium 69mg, Carbohydrate 63.4g, Fiber 5.4g, Sugars 17.3g, Protein 9.3g, Potassium 577mg

Quinoa And Oats

Preparation time: 10 minutes | Cooking time: 7 hours | Servings: 6

Ingredients:
- 2 tablespoons stevia
- 2 tablespoons maple syrup
- ½ cup quinoa
- ½ teaspoon vanilla extract
- 1 and ½ cups steel cut oats
- 4 cups water

Directions:
1. In your slow cooker, mix the oats with the quinoa, water, stevia, maple syrup and vanilla, cover and cook on Low for 7 hours.
2. Stir the oatmeal, divide it into bowls and serve.

Nutrition: Calories 148, Fat 2.2g, Cholesterol 0mg, Sodium 7mg, Carbohydrate 32.4g, Fiber 3.1g, Sugars 4.2g, Protein 4.7g, Potassium 170mg

Radish and Eggs Mix

Preparation time: 10 minutes | Cooking time: 2 hours | Servings: 4

Ingredients:
- 2 spring onions, chopped
- 1 cup radishes, cubed
- 8 eggs, whisked
- ½ cup non-fat milk
- ½ teaspoon turmeric powder
- ½ teaspoon garam masala
- A pinch of black pepper

Directions:
1. In the slow cooker, combine the spring onions with the eggs, radishes and the other ingredients, put the lid on and cook on High for 2 hours.
2. Divide the mix into bowls and serve for breakfast.

Nutrition: Calories 145, Fat .8.8g, Cholesterol 328mg, Sodium 153mg, Carbohydrate 4.1g, Fiber 0.7g, Sugars 2.9g, Protein 12.4g, Potassium 264mg

Pumpkin Oatmeal

Preparation time: 10 minutes | Cooking time: 9 hours | Servings: 4

Ingredients:
- 1 cup steel cut oats
- 2 tablespoons stevia
- ½ teaspoon cinnamon powder
- A pinch of cloves, ground
- ½ cup pumpkin puree
- 4 cups water
- Olive oil cooking spray
- ½ cup fat-free milk
- A pinch of nutmeg, ground
- A pinch of allspice, ground
- A pinch of ginger, ground

Directions:
1. Grease your slow cooker with the cooking spray, add the oats, the pumpkin puree, water, milk, stevia, cinnamon, cloves, allspice, ginger and nutmeg, cover and cook on Low for 9 hours.
2. Stir the oatmeal, divide it into bowls and serve.

Nutrition: Calories 100, Fat 1.5g, Cholesterol 1mg, Sodium 26mg, Carbohydrate 25.5g, Fiber 3g,

Sugars 2.7g, Protein 4g, Potassium 189mg

Raspberry Oatmeal

Preparation time: 10 minutes | Cooking time: 6 hours | Servings: 4

Ingredients:
- 1 tablespoon coconut oil
- 1 cup raspberries
- 4 tablespoons walnuts
- 2 cups water
- 1 cup nonfat milk
- 1 tablespoon stevia
- 1 cup steel cut oats
- ½ teaspoon vanilla extract

Directions:
1. In your slow cooker, combine the oil with the oats, water, milk, stevia, vanilla, raspberries and walnuts, cover and cook on Low for 6 hours.
2. Divide the oatmeal into bowls and serve.

Nutrition: Calories 195, Fat 9.5g, Cholesterol 1mg, Sodium 38mg, Carbohydrate 28.9g, Fiber 4.6g, Sugars 4.7g, Protein 6.9g, Potassium 258mg

Peppers Eggs Mix

Preparation time: 10 minutes | Cooking time: 2 hours and 30 minutes | Servings: 4

Ingredients:
- 8 eggs, whisked
- 1 cup red roasted peppers, chopped
- 2 spring onions, chopped
- 1 teaspoon oregano, dried
- 1 teaspoon chili powder
- 1 teaspoon rosemary, dried
- ½ cup coconut cream
- A pinch of black pepper

Directions:
1. In the slow cooker, combine the eggs with the peppers, spring onions and the other ingredients, toss, put the lid on and cook on High for 2 hours and 30 minutes.
2. Divide the mix between plates and serve for breakfast.

Nutrition: Calories 272, Fat .20.1g, Cholesterol 327mg, Sodium 816mg, Carbohydrate 11.7g, Fiber 1.4g, Sugars 7.9g, Protein 12g, Potassium 240mg

Delicious Frittata

Preparation time: 10 minutes | Cooking time: 3 hours | Servings: 6

Ingredients:
- A pinch of black pepper
- 14 ounces small artichoke hearts, drained
- ¼ cup green onions, chopped
- 12 ounces roasted red peppers, chopped
- 4 ounces low-fat cheese, grated
- 8 eggs, whisked

Directions:
1. In your slow cooker, mix the eggs with the red peppers, artichokes, green onions and black pepper and whisk.
2. Spread the cheese all over, cover and cook on Low for 3 hours.
3. Slice, divide between plates and serve.

Nutrition: Calories 201, Fat 12.2g, Cholesterol 238mg, Sodium 526mg, Carbohydrate 9g, Fiber 2.8g, Sugars 3.1g, Protein 14.2g, Potassium 203mg

Spinach Frittata

Preparation time: 10 minutes | Cooking time: 2 hours | Servings: 4

Ingredients:
- A pinch of white pepper
- 1 tablespoon olive oil
- ½ cup yellow onion, chopped
- 1 cup low-fat cheese, shredded
- 1 cup baby spinach leaves
- 1 tomato, chopped
- 3 egg whites
- 3 eggs
- 2 tablespoon low-fat milk
- A pinch of black pepper

Directions:
1. In a bowl, mix the eggs with the egg whites, milk, white and black pepper, spinach and tomato and stir.
2. Grease the slow cooker with the oil, pour eggs mix, spread the cheese on top, cover and cook on Low for 2 hours.
3. Slice the frittata, divide between plates and serve.

Nutrition: Calories 217, Fat 16.3g, Cholesterol 153mg, Sodium 272mg, Carbohydrate 3.4g, Fiber 0.7g, Sugars 2g, Protein 14.7g, Potassium 224mg

Potato and Shrimp Bowls

Preparation time: 10 minutes | Cooking time: 3 hours | Servings: 4

Ingredients:
- 8 eggs, whisked
- ½ pound gold potatoes, peeled and cubed
- 2 tablespoons parsley, chopped
- ½ pound shrimp, peeled and deveined
- 1 teaspoon turmeric powder
- ½ cup low-sodium veggie stock
- A pinch of black pepper

Directions:
1. In the slow cooker, combine the potatoes

with the other ingredients except the shrimp, put the lid on and cook on High for 2 hours and 30 minutes.
2. Add the shrimp, cook the mix on High for 30 minutes more, divide into bowls and serve for breakfast.

Nutrition: Calories 236, Fat .9.8g, Cholesterol 447mg, Sodium 312mg, Carbohydrate 11.6g, Fiber 1.7g, Sugars 1.6g, Protein 24.8g, Potassium 473mg

Breakfast Veggie Omelet

Preparation time: 10 minutes | Cooking time: 2 hours | Servings: 4

Ingredients:
- 1 red bell pepper, chopped
- Black pepper to the taste
- 1 cup broccoli florets
- A pinch of chili powder
- A pinch of garlic powder
- 1 yellow onion, chopped
- Cooking spray
- 6 eggs, whisked
- ½ cup low-fat milk
- 1 garlic clove, minced

Directions:
1. In a bowl, mix the eggs with the milk, black pepper, chili powder, garlic powder, red bell pepper, broccoli, onion and garlic and whisk well.
2. Grease your slow cooker with the cooking spray, spread the eggs mix on the bottom, cover and cook on High for 2 hours.
3. Slice the omelet, divide it between plates and serve.

Nutrition: Calories 171, Fat 8.7g, Cholesterol 247mg, Sodium 396mg, Carbohydrate 13g, Fiber 1.8g, Sugars 7.5g, Protein 10.9g, Potassium 308mg

Scrambled Eggs

Preparation time: 10 minutes | Cooking time: 8 hours | Servings: 8

Ingredients:
- 16 ounces low-fat cheese, shredded
- 12 eggs
- 6 ounces hash browns
- ½ tablespoon cayenne powder
- 15 ounces sausage, sliced
- 1 cup nonfat milk
- Black pepper to the taste

Directions:
1. In a bowl, mix the eggs with the hash browns, sausage, milk, black pepper and cayenne and whisk well.
2. Spread this into your slow cooker, spread the cheese on top, cover and cook on Low for 8 hours.
3. Stir the scrambled eggs, divide them between plates and serve.

Nutrition: Calories 588, Fat 43.9g, Cholesterol 350mg, Sodium 1072mg, Carbohydrate 12.5g, Fiber 0.8g, Sugars 3.8g, Protein 34.6g, Potassium 477mg

Cilantro Hash

Preparation time: 10 minutes | Cooking time: 4 hours | Servings: 4

Ingredients:
- 1 pound hash browns
- 2 spring onions, chopped
- 1 cup cherry tomatoes, halved
- 4 eggs, whisked
- A pinch of cayenne pepper
- ½ cup low-sodium veggie stock
- 1 tablespoon cilantro, chopped

Directions:
1. In the slow cooker, combine the hash browns with the eggs and the other ingredients, put the lid on and cook on Low for 4 hours.
2. Divide the hash into bowls and serve right away for breakfast.

Nutrition: Calories 376, Fat .18.7g, Cholesterol 164mg, Sodium 502mg, Carbohydrate 43g, Fiber 4.4g, Sugars 3.5g, Protein 9.5g, Potassium 842mg

Apple And Raisins Oatmeal

Preparation time: 10 minutes | Cooking time: 6 hours | Servings: 4

Ingredients:
- 2 cups almond milk
- ½ teaspoon cinnamon powder
- 1 tablespoon low-fat butter
- 2 tablespoons stevia
- 2 drops vanilla extract
- Cooking spray
- 1 cup apple, chopped
- ¼ cup raisins
- 1 cup old-fashioned oats

Directions:
1. Grease your slow cooker with the cooking spray, add milk, stevia, butter, cinnamon and vanilla and stir.
2. Add oats, apples and raisins, cover and cook on Low for 7 hours.
3. Divide into bowls and serve.

Nutrition: Calories 437, Fat 43.9g, Cholesterol 350mg, Sodium 1072mg, Carbohydrate 12.5g, Fiber 0.8g, Sugars 3.8g, Protein 34.6g, Potassium 477mg

Delicious Peanut Butter Oats

Preparation time: 10 minutes | Cooking time: 6 hours | Servings: 2

Ingredients:
- 2 tablespoon chia seeds
- 4 tablespoons peanut butter
- 1 cup rolled oats
- 1 cup almond milk
- 1 tablespoon stevia

Directions:
1. In your slow cooker, mix the oats with the milk, chia, peanut butter and stevia, cover and cook on Low for 6 hours.
2. Stir the oats mix, divide into bowls and serve.

Nutrition: Calories 334, Fat 25.5g, Cholesterol 0mg, Sodium 85mg, Carbohydrate 29.9, Fiber 6.1g, Sugars 3.7g, Protein 8.9g, Potassium 356mg

Black Beans and Eggs Salad

Preparation time: 10 minutes | Cooking time: 4 hours | Servings: 4

Ingredients:
- 8 eggs, whisked
- 4 spring onions, chopped
- 1 teaspoon chili powder
- ½ teaspoon smoked paprika
- ½ cup low-sodium veggie stock
- A pinch of black pepper
- 1 cup kalamata olives, pitted and halved
- 1 and ½ cups canned black beans, no-salt-added, drained and rinsed

Directions:
1. In the slow cooker, combine the eggs with the spring onions, black beans and the other ingredients, toss, put the lid on and cook on Low for 4 hours.
2. Divide the mix into bowls and serve for breakfast.

Nutrition: Calories 422, Fat .13.5g, Cholesterol 327mg, Sodium 446mg, Carbohydrate 50g, Fiber 12.9g, Sugars 2.8g, Protein 27.5g, Potassium 1260mg

Orange And Strawberry Breakfast Mix

Preparation time: 5 minutes | Cooking time: 4 hours | Servings: 2

Ingredients:
- 1 cup low-fat milk
- 20 ounces strawberries
- 1 cup orange juice
- 6 ounces low-fat yogurt

Directions:
1. In your slow cooker, mix orange juice with milk and strawberries, cover and cook on Low for 4 hours.
2. Divide the yogurt into bowls, add the orange and strawberry mix on top and serve.

Nutrition: Calories 258, Fat 33g, Cholesterol 11mg, Sodium 117mg, Carbohydrate 46.8g, Fiber 5.9g, Sugars 36.6g, Protein 11.7g, Potassium 1064mg

Omelet

Preparation time: 10 minutes | Cooking time: 2 hours | Servings: 4

Ingredients:
- 8 eggs, whisked
- 2 ounces low-fat cheddar cheese, grated
- 2 cups spinach, torn
- Cooking spray
- 2 tablespoons chives, chopped
- A pinch of cayenne pepper
- Salt and black pepper to the taste
- For the red pepper relish:
- 2 tablespoons green onion, chopped
- 1 tablespoon vinegar
- 1 cup red pepper, chopped

Directions:
1. In a bowl, mix eggs with salt, pepper, cayenne and chives and stir well.
2. Grease your slow cooker with cooking spray, add eggs mix and spread.
3. Add spinach and cheese, toss, cover and cook on High for 2 hours.
4. In a bowl, mix red pepper with green onions, black pepper to the taste and the vinegar and stir well.
5. Slice the omelet, divide it between plates, top with the relish and serve for breakfast.

Nutrition: Calories 200, Fat 13.8g, Cholesterol 342mg, Sodium 225mg, Carbohydrate 46g, Fiber 0.9g, Sugars 2.4g, Protein 15.4g, Potassium 288mg

Orange Hash Mix

Preparation time: 10 minutes | Cooking time: 3 hours | Servings: 4

Ingredients:
- 1 pound hash browns
- 1 cup cherry tomatoes, halved
- 1 orange, peeled and cut into segments
- 1 tablespoon orange juice
- 1 and ½ teaspoon turmeric powder
- ½ cup low-sodium veggie stock
- A pinch of cayenne pepper

Directions:
1. In the slow cooker, combine the hash browns with the tomatoes, orange segments and the other ingredients, put the lid on and cook on

High for 3 hours.
2. Divide into bowls and serve for breakfast.

Nutrition: Calories 322, Fat .14.4g, Cholesterol 0mg, Sodium 439mg, Carbohydrate 44.7g, Fiber 4.4g, Sugars 4.8g, Protein 4g, Potassium 818mg

Fruits and Cereals Mix

Preparation time: 10 minutes | Cooking time: 6 hours | Servings: 6

Ingredients:
- ½ cup whole wheat and barley cereals
- 4 cups mixed orange, apple, grapes and pineapple pieces
- 12 ounces almond milk
- 2 tablespoons stevia
- ¼ cup coconut, toasted and shredded

Directions:
1. In your slow cooker, mix the fruits with the stevia, cereals and milk, cover and cook on Low for 6 hours.
2. Divide into bowls, sprinkle coconut on top and serve.

Nutrition: Calories 228, Fat 14.9g, Cholesterol 0mg, Sodium 56mg, Carbohydrate 30.8g, Fiber 6g, Sugars 13.3g, Protein 2.6g, Potassium 195mg

Breakfast Berries Compote

Preparation time: 10 minutes | Cooking time: 4 hours | Servings: 4

Ingredients:
- 2 tablespoons white wine vinegar
- 2 tablespoons lemon juice
- 2 cups blueberries
- ½ cup palm sugar
- 2 peaches, pitted, peeled and cut into wedges
- ½ teaspoon lemon zest, grated
- 1 and ½ cups blackberries
- 1 and ½ cups raspberries

Directions:
1. In your slow cooker, mix blueberries with sugar, vinegar, lemon juice and lemon zest, cover and cook on Low for 4 hours.
2. Divide this into 4 bowl, top with raspberries, blackberries and peach wedges and serve for breakfast.

Nutrition: Calories 273, Fat 0.9g, Cholesterol 0mg, Sodium 1831mg, Carbohydrate 61.9g, Fiber 6g, Sugars 54.2g, Protein 1.8g, Potassium 1857mg

Shrimp and Eggs

Preparation time: 10 minutes | Cooking time: 2 hours | Servings: 2

Ingredients:
- 8 eggs, whisked
- 1 and ½ cups shrimp, cooked, peeled, deveined and cubed
- ½ cup spring onions, chopped
- 1 teaspoon turmeric powder
- ½ teaspoon sweet paprika
- ¼ cup almond milk
- A pinch of black pepper
- 1 tablespoon chives, chopped

Directions:
1. In the slow cooker, combine the eggs with the shrimp, spring onions and the other ingredients, put the lid on and cook on High for 2 hours.
2. Divide the mix between plates and serve for breakfast.

Nutrition: Calories 242, Fat .13.5g, Cholesterol 459mg, Sodium 280mg, Carbohydrate 3.9g, Fiber 0.9g, Sugars 1.5g, Protein 26g, Potassium 320mg

Apples and Dates Oatmeal

Preparation time: 10 minutes | Cooking time: 7 hours | Servings: 4

Ingredients:
- 1 cup dates, dried and chopped
- 1 cup walnuts, chopped
- 4 cups water
- 3 cups rolled oats
- 1 teaspoon cloves, ground
- 1 tablespoon ginger, ground
- 1 teaspoon turmeric powder
- 3 cups whole grain cereal flakes
- 1 cup apples, dried and chopped
- 2 tablespoons cinnamon powder
- 1 cup coconut sugar

Directions:
1. In your slow cooker, mix the water with the oats, cereal flakes, apples, dates, walnuts, cinnamon, sugar, cloves, ginger and turmeric, cover and cook on Low for 7 hours.
2. Divide into bowls and serve.

Nutrition: Calories 946, Fat 24.6g, Cholesterol 0mg, Sodium 658mg, Carbohydrate 168.8g, Fiber 23.7g, Sugars 57.7g, Protein 23.9g, Potassium 1077mg

Sweet Rice Bowls

Preparation time: 10 minutes | Cooking time: 2 hours and 30 minutes | Servings: 4

Ingredients:
- 2 cups almond milk
- 2 teaspoons maple syrups
- 2 teaspoons sugar
- 1 cup white rice
- ½ teaspoon almond extract
- ½ teaspoon nutmeg, ground

Directions:

1. In the slow cooker, combine the milk with the rice, sugar and the other ingredients, put the lid on and cook on High for 2 hours and 30 minutes.
2. Divide into bowls and serve for breakfast.

Nutrition: Calories 464, Fat .29g, Cholesterol 0mg, Sodium 21mg, Carbohydrate 48.1g, Fiber 3.3g, Sugars 8.2g, Protein 6.1g, Potassium 377mg

Scrambled Eggs and Veggies

Preparation time: 10 minutes | Cooking time: 8 hours | Servings: 4

Ingredients:

- A pinch of black pepper
- A splash of hot pepper
- 3 eggs
- ¼ cup green bell pepper, chopped
- Cooking spray
- ¾ cup tomato, chopped
- ¼ cup green onions, chopped
- ¼ cup fat-free milk

Directions:

1. In a bowl, mix the eggs with the bell pepper, tomato, onions, milk, black pepper and hot pepper and stir.
2. Grease the slow cooker with the cooking spray, add eggs mix, cover and cook on Low for 8 hours.
3. Stir the eggs, divide them between plates and serve.

Nutrition: Calories 69, Fat 3.6g, Cholesterol 123mg, Sodium 58mg, Carbohydrate 4.3g, Fiber 0.9g, Sugars 3g, Protein 5.4g, Potassium 216mg

Mexican Casserole

Preparation time: 10 minutes | Cooking time: 4 hours | Servings: 8

Ingredients:

- 2 garlic cloves, minced
- 3 egg whites
- 2 tablespoons whole wheat flour
- ¾ cup tomato passata
- 15 ounces canned black beans, drained and rinsed
- 8 ounces canned green chili peppers, chopped
- ½ cup green onions, chopped
- Cooking spray
- 1 cup low-fat cheddar cheese, grated
- 3 egg yolks
- A splash of hot pepper sauce
- ½ cup fat-free milk
- 1 tablespoon cilantro, chopped

green onions, pepper sauce, salt, garlic and cheese.
2. In a bowl, beat egg whites with a mixer.
3. In a separate bowl, mix egg yolks with salt and flour and whisk well.
4. Add egg whites, milk and cilantro and whisk well again.
5. Pour this over beans mix, spread well, cover and cook on Low for 4 hours.
6. Slice, divide between plates and serve for breakfast.

Nutrition: Calories 381, Fat 8.9g, Cholesterol 94mg, Sodium 159mg, Carbohydrate 58.1g, Fiber 16.5g, Sugars 15g, Protein 21.6g, Potassium 1406mg

Quinoa and Tomato Bowls

Preparation time: 10 minutes | Cooking time: 2 hours | Servings: 4

Ingredients:

- 2 cups low-sodium veggie stock
- ½ cup scallions, chopped
- 1 cup cherry tomatoes, halved
- 1 and ½ cups quinoa
- A pinch of black pepper

Directions:

1. In your slow cooker, combine the quinoa with the tomatoes and the other ingredients, put the lid on and cook on Low for 2 hours.
2. Divide into bowls and serve for breakfast.

Nutrition: Calories 254, Fat .4g, Cholesterol 0mg, Sodium 78mg, Carbohydrate 44.6g, Fiber 5.3g, Sugars 2g, Protein 9.6g, Potassium 500mg

Shrimp Frittata

Preparation time: 10 minutes | Cooking time: 4 hours | Servings: 4

Ingredients:

- 8 cherry tomatoes, halved
- 1 tablespoon parsley, chopped
- 4 ounces shrimp, peeled, deveined and cut into halves horizontally
- A pinch of black pepper
- A pinch of garlic powder
- 2 eggs
- 4 ounces canned artichokes, drained and chopped
- ¼ cup fat-free milk
- ¼ cup green onions, chopped
- Cooking spray
- 3 tablespoons low-fat cheddar cheese, grated

stir well.
2. Grease your slow cooker with the cooking spray, add eggs mix, cover and cook on Low for 3 hours and 30 minutes.
3. Add shrimp, artichokes, cheddar cheese, tomatoes and parsley on top, cover and cook on Low for 30 minutes.
4. Divide frittata between plates and serve for breakfast.

Nutrition: Calories 154, Fat 5.1g, Cholesterol 147mg, Sodium 181mg, Carbohydrate 14.6g, Fiber 4.7g, Sugars 7.9g, Protein 14.3g, Potassium 818mg

Tofu Scramble

Preparation time: 10 minutes | Cooking time: 5 hours | Servings: 4

Ingredients:
- 1 teaspoon chili powder
- ½ teaspoon oregano, dried
- ½ teaspoon cumin, ground
- 18 ounces package firm tofu, drained well, pat dried and crumbled
- 2 poblano chili peppers, chopped
- 2 garlic cloves, minced
- ½ cup onion, chopped
- 2 tomatoes, peeled and chopped
- 1 tablespoon olive oil
- 1 tablespoon lime juice
- 1 tablespoon cilantro, chopped

Directions:
1. Grease the slow cooker with the oil and add chili peppers, garlic and onion.
2. Also add chili powder, oregano and cumin and stir.
3. Add tofu, tomatoes, lime juice and cilantro, stir well again, cover and cook on Low for 5 hours.
4. Divide the scramble between plates and serve.

Nutrition: Calories 152, Fat 9.2g, Cholesterol 0mg, Sodium 28mg, Carbohydrate 9.4g, Fiber 2.9g, Sugars 4.3g, Protein 11.9g, Potassium 464mg

Eggs and Corn Mix

Preparation time: 10 minutes | Cooking time: 2 hours | Servings: 4

Ingredients:
- 8 eggs, whisked
- 1 cup corn
- ½ cup coconut cream
- A pinch of cayenne pepper
- ½ teaspoon turmeric powder
- ½ teaspoon rosemary, dried
- ½ teaspoon coriander, ground

Directions:
1. In your slow cooker, combine the eggs with the corn, cream and the other ingredients, toss, put the lid on and cook on High for 2 hours.
2. Divide into bowls and serve for breakfast.

Nutrition: Calories 230, Fat .6.4g, Cholesterol 327mg, Sodium 134mg, Carbohydrate 9.9g, Fiber 1.9g, Sugars 3g, Protein 13.1g, Potassium 311mg

Squash and Apples Breakfast Mix

Preparation time: 10 minutes | Cooking time: 6 hours | Servings: 2

Ingredients:
- 1 big apple, cored, peeled and cut into wedges
- 2 teaspoons avocado oil
- 1 acorn squash, halved, deseeded and cubed
- 2 tablespoons stevia

Directions:
1. Grease your slow cooker with the oil, add apple, squash and stevia, toss, cover and cook on Low for 6 hours.
2. Divide into bowls and serve for breakfast.

Nutrition: Calories 150, Fat 1g, Cholesterol 0mg, Sodium 8mg, Carbohydrate 53.1g, Fiber 6.1g, Sugars 11.6g, Protein 2.1g, Potassium 882mg

Raisin Rice Bowls

Preparation time: 10 minutes | Cooking time: 3 hours | Servings: 4

Ingredients:
- 1 cup white rice
- 2 cups almond milk
- ½ cup raisins
- ½ teaspoon cinnamon powder
- ¼ tablespoon sugar
- 2 tablespoons walnuts, chopped

Directions:
1. In the slow cooker, mix the rice with the raisins, milk and the other ingredients, toss, put the lid on and cook on Low for 3 hours.
2. Divide the mix into bowls and serve for breakfast.

Nutrition: Calories 526, Fat .31.3g, Cholesterol 0mg, Sodium 22mg, Carbohydrate 59.1g, Fiber 4.2g, Sugars 15.6g, Protein 7.6g, Potassium 525mg

Corn Pudding

Preparation time: 10 minutes | Cooking time: 6 hours | Servings: 8

Ingredients:
- 2 cups cornmeal
- A pinch of nutmeg,

ground
- 3 cups fat-free milk
- ¼ cup maple syrup
- ¼ teaspoon cinnamon powder
- A pinch of cloves, ground
- 3 cups water
- ½ cup raisins
- A pinch of ginger, grated

Directions:
1. In your slow cooker, mix the water with the milk and cornmeal and stir.
2. Add raisins, maple syrup, nutmeg, cinnamon, cloves and ginger, stir, cover, cook on Low for 6 hours.
3. Divide between plates and serve.

Nutrition: Calories 197, Fat 1.2g, Cholesterol 2mg, Sodium 64mg, Carbohydrate 41.8g, Fiber 2.6g, Sugars 15.9g, Protein 5.8g, Potassium 320mg

Sweet Potatoes Mix

Preparation time: 10 minutes | Cooking time: 7 hours | Servings: 8

Ingredients:
- 1 tablespoon olive oil
- 2 tablespoons stevia
- 4 sweet potatoes, peeled and cut into wedges
- Black pepper to the taste
- ¼ cup water
- A pinch of rosemary, dried

Directions:
1. In your slow cooker, mix the potatoes with the oil, black pepper, rosemary, water and stevia, toss, cover and cook on Low for 7 hours.
2. Divide between plates and serve for breakfast.

Nutrition: Calories 120, Fat 2.6g, Cholesterol 0mg, Sodium 147mg, Carbohydrate 26.8g, Fiber 3.2g, Sugars 1.5g, Protein 1.3g, Potassium 612mg

Shrimp Salad

Preparation time: 10 minutes | Cooking time: 1 hour | Servings: 4

Ingredients:
- 1 pound shrimp, peeled and deveined
- 1 cup corn
- 1 cup baby spinach
- 1 cup cherry tomatoes, halved
- 1 teaspoon chili powder
- ½ cup low-sodium veggie stock
- 1 tablespoon cilantro, chopped

Directions:
1. In your slow cooker, combine the shrimp with the corn, spinach and the other ingredients, put the lid on and cook on High for 1 hour.

2. Divide into bowls and serve for breakfast.

Nutrition: Calories 182, Fat .2.6g, Cholesterol 239mg, Sodium 346mg, Carbohydrate 11.9g, Fiber 2g, Sugars 2.6g, Protein 27.8g, Potassium 458mg

Almond and Cherries Oats

Preparation time: 10 minutes | Cooking time: 8 hours | Servings: 4

Ingredients:
- 2 cups almond milk
- 2 tablespoons cocoa powder
- ¼ cup stevia
- 1 cup steel cut oats
- 2 cups water
- ½ teaspoon almond extract
- 1/3 cup cherries, dried

Directions:
1. In your slow cooker, mix almond milk with oats, water, dried cherries, cocoa powder, stevia and the almond extract, stir, cover and cook on Low for 8 hours.
2. Divide the oats into bowls and serve for breakfast.

Nutrition: Calories 390, Fat 30.3g, Cholesterol 0mg, Sodium 28mg, Carbohydrate 44g, Fiber 5.7g, Sugars 4.3g, Protein 6g, Potassium 486mg

Cranberry Toast

Preparation time: 10 minutes | Cooking time: 5 hours | Servings: 4

Ingredients:
- 4 whole wheat bread slices, cubed
- 1 tablespoon coconut oil
- 1 tablespoon chia seeds
- ½ tablespoon stevia
- ½ teaspoon vanilla extract
- ½ teaspoon cinnamon powder
- 1 cup almond milk

Directions:
1. Add coconut oil to your slow cooker, also add bread cubes and toss them.
2. Also add milk, chia, vanilla, stevia and cinnamon, toss, cover, cook on Low for 5 hours, divide into bowls and serve for breakfast.

Nutrition: Calories 262, Fat 20.2g, Cholesterol 0mg, Sodium 142mg, Carbohydrate 20.1g, Fiber 4.9g, Sugars 3.6g, Protein 5.8g, Potassium 248mg

Strawberry and Chia Bowls

Preparation time: 10 minutes | Cooking time: 2

- 3 tablespoons chia seeds
- 1 cup non-fat milk
- ½ teaspoon vanilla extract
- ¼ teaspoon almond extract
- ½ cup non-fat yogurt

Directions:
1. In your slow cooker, mix the berries with the chia seeds and the other ingredients, put the lid on and cook on Low for 2 hours.
2. Divide into bowls and serve for breakfast.

Nutrition: Calories 136, Fat 3.2g, Cholesterol 3mg, Sodium 95mg, Carbohydrate 21.3g, Fiber 4.8g, Sugars 8.7g, Protein 5.3g, Potassium 136mg

Burrito Bowls

Preparation time: 10 minutes | Cooking time: 6 hours | Servings: 8

Ingredients:
- 3 cups spinach leaves, torn
- 16 ounces tofu, crumbled
- 1 green bell pepper, chopped
- A pinch of black pepper
- ¼ cup scallions, chopped
- 15 ounces canned black beans, drained and rinsed
- ¼ teaspoon cumin, ground
- ½ teaspoon turmeric powder
- ½ teaspoon sweet paprika
- 1 cup tomato sauce, sodium free
- ½ cup water
- ¼ teaspoon chili powder

Directions:
1. In your slow cooker, mix tofu with bell pepper, scallions, black beans, salsa, water, cumin, turmeric, paprika, salt, pepper and chili powder, stir, cover and cook on Low for 6 hours.
2. Add spinach, toss well, divide into bowls and serve for breakfast.

Nutrition: Calories 238, Fat 3.3g, Cholesterol 0mg, Sodium 181mg, Carbohydrate 37.8g, Fiber 9.7g, Sugars 3.7g, Protein 17.1g, Potassium 1083mg

Spiced Coconut Oats

Preparation time: 10 minutes | Cooking time: 4 hours | Servings: 6

Ingredients:
- 1 tablespoon flax seed, ground
- 2 teaspoons vanilla extract
- 2 teaspoons stevia
- 2 apples, cored, peeled and chopped
- ½ teaspoon cinnamon powder
- ¼ teaspoon nutmeg, ground
- 1 and ½ cups water
- 1 and ½ cups coconut milk
- 1 cup steel cut oats
- ¼ teaspoon allspice, ground
- ¼ teaspoon ginger powder

Directions:
1. Spray your slow cooker with cooking spray, add apple pieces, milk, water, cinnamon, oats, allspice, nutmeg, cardamom, ginger, vanilla, flax seeds and stevia, cover and cook on Low for 4 hours.
2. Stir the oatmeal, divide into bowls and serve for breakfast.

Nutrition: Calories 103, Fat 1.6g, Cholesterol 0mg, Sodium 4mg, Carbohydrate 20.4g, Fiber 3.6g, Sugars 8.1g, Protein 2.2g, Potassium 145mg

Apples and Apricots Bowls

Preparation time: 10 minutes | Cooking time: 2 hours | Servings: 4

Ingredients:
- ½ pound peaches, pitted and cut into wedges
- ½ pound apricots, cubed
- ½ cup coconut cream
- 2 tablespoons maple syrup
- 2 tablespoons non-fat butter

Directions:
1. In your slow cooker, mix the peaches with the apricots and the other ingredients, put the lid on and cook on High for 2 hours.
2. Divide into bowls and serve for breakfast.

Nutrition: Calories 170, Fat 7.6g, Cholesterol 3mg, Sodium 234mg, Carbohydrate 19.3g, Fiber 2.1g, Sugars 13.8g, Protein 8.6g, Potassium 282mg

Carrot Oatmeal

Preparation time: 10 minutes | Cooking time: 7 hours | Servings: 4

Ingredients:
- 1 teaspoon cardamom, ground
- ½ teaspoon stevia
- 2 cups coconut milk
- ½ cup steel cut oats
- A pinch of saffron powder
- Cooking spray
- 1 cup carrots, shredded

Directions:
1. Spray your slow cooker with cooking spray, add milk, oats, carrots, cardamom and stevia, stir, cover and cook on Low for 7 hours.
2. Stir oatmeal, divide into bowls, sprinkle saffron on top and serve for breakfast.

Nutrition: Calories 329, Fat 29.5g, Cholesterol 0mg, Sodium 38mg, Carbohydrate 24.1g, Fiber 4.5g, Sugars 5.5g, Protein 4.4g, Potassium 446mg

Blueberries Oatmeal

Preparation time: 10 minutes | Cooking time: 8 hours | Servings: 4

Ingredients:
- 1 cup coconut milk
- 1 cup blueberries
- 2 tablespoons stevia
- ½ teaspoon vanilla extract
- 1 cup steel cut oats
- Coconut flakes for serving
- Cooking spray

Directions:
1. Spray your slow cooker with cooking spray, add oats, milk, stevia, vanilla and blueberries, toss, cover and cook on Low for 8 hours.
2. Divide the oatmeal into bowls, sprinkle coconut flakes on top and serve.

Nutrition: Calories 590, Fat 49.1g, Cholesterol 0mg, Sodium 30mg, Carbohydrate 37.8g, Fiber 13.2g, Sugars 12g, Protein 7.7g, Potassium 614mg

Orange and Avocado Quinoa

Preparation time: 10 minutes | Cooking time: 2 hours | Servings: 4

Ingredients:
- 1 cup quinoa
- 1 and ½ cups almond milk
- 1 orange, peeled and cut into segments
- 1 avocado, peeled, pitted and cubed
- 1 tablespoon maple syrup
- 1 teaspoon cinnamon powder
- ½ teaspoon almond extract

Directions:
1. In your slow cooker, combine the quinoa with the milk, orange and the other ingredients, put the lid on and cook on High for 2 hours.
2. Toss the mix, divide into bowls and serve.

Nutrition: Calories 502, Fat 33.9g, Cholesterol 0mg, Sodium 19mg, Carbohydrate 45.4g, Fiber 9.4g, Sugars 10.6g, Protein 9.4g, Potassium 814mg

Tofu and Veggies Frittata

Preparation time: 10 minutes | Cooking time: 6 hours | Servings: 4

Ingredients:
- 3 tablespoons garlic, minced
- 1 red bell pepper, chopped
- 1 pound firm tofu, drained, pressed and crumbled
- 2 tablespoons olive oil
- 1 yellow onion, chopped
- ¼ teaspoon turmeric powder
- 1 teaspoon basil, dried
- 1 teaspoon oregano, dried
- 1 tablespoon lemon juice
- ½ cup kalamata olives, pitted and halved
- Black pepper to the taste

Directions:
1. Add the oil to your slow cooker and spread the crumbled tofu.
2. Add onion, turmeric, garlic, bell pepper, olives, basil, oregano, lemon juice and pepper, toss a bit, cover and cook on Low for 6 hours.
3. Divide frittata between plates and serve for breakfast.

Nutrition: Calories 224, Fat 15.2g, Cholesterol 0mg, Sodium 444mg, Carbohydrate 14.5g, Fiber 3g, Sugars 5.8g, Protein 10.8g, Potassium 306mg

Coconut Hash Bowls

Preparation time: 10 minutes | Cooking time: 4 hours | Servings: 4

Ingredients:
- 1 pound hash browns
- 1 cup coconut cream
- 1 tablespoon oregano, chopped
- 1 tablespoon basil, chopped
- 1 teaspoon chili powder
- 1 teaspoon sweet paprika
- 6 eggs, whisked
- A pinch of cayenne pepper

Directions:
1. In your slow cooker, combine the hash browns with the cream, oregano and the other ingredients, put the lid on and cook on Low for 4 hours.
2. Divide between plates and serve for breakfast.

Nutrition: Calories 540, Fat 35.4g, Cholesterol 246mg, Sodium 496mg, Carbohydrate 45.1g, Fiber 5.9g, Sugars 4.4g, Protein 13.4g, Potassium 946mg

Chia Pudding

Preparation time: 10 minutes | Cooking time: 2 hours | Servings: 4

Ingredients:
- ½ cup coconut chia granola
- 2 tablespoons coconut, shredded and unsweetened
- 2 teaspoons cocoa powder
- ½ teaspoon vanilla extract
- ½ cup chia seeds
- 2 cups coconut milk
- ¼ cup maple syrup
- ½ teaspoon cinnamon powder

Directions:
1. In your slow cooker, mix chia granola with chia seeds, coconut milk, coconut, maple

syrup, cinnamon, cocoa powder and vanilla, toss, cover and cook on High for 2 hours.
2. Divide chia pudding into bowls and serve for breakfast.

Nutrition: Calories 482, Fat 37.6g, Cholesterol 0mg, Sodium 32mg, Carbohydrate 32.5g, Fiber 11g, Sugars 17.5g, Protein 7.1g, Potassium 492mg

Breakfast Potatoes

Preparation time: 10 minutes | Cooking time: 4 hours | Servings: 8

Ingredients:
- 12 ounces coconut milk
- 1 cup tofu, crumbled
- Cooking spray
- 1 tablespoons parsley, chopped
- 2 pounds gold potatoes, halved and sliced
- 1 yellow onion, cut into medium wedges
- Black pepper to the taste

Directions:
1. Coat your slow cooker with cooking spray and arrange half of the potatoes on the bottom.
2. Layer half of the onion wedges and half of the coconut milk, tofu and pepper.
3. Add the rest of the potatoes, onion wedges, coconut milk, tofu and stock, cover and cook on High for 4 hours.
4. Sprinkle parsley on top, divide the whole mix between plates and serve.

Nutrition: Calories 218, Fat 12.3g, Cholesterol 0mg, Sodium 151mg, Carbohydrate 24.5g, Fiber 4.6g, Sugars 4.8g, Protein 5.4g, Potassium 650mg

Nutmeg Oatmeal

Preparation time: 10 minutes | Cooking time: 2 hours | Servings: 4

Ingredients:
- 1 cup old fashioned oats
- 2 cups non-fat milk
- 1 tablespoon sugar
- 1 teaspoon nutmeg, ground
- 1 teaspoon cinnamon powder
- 1 teaspoon vanilla extract3

Directions:
1. In your slow cooker, combine the oats with the milk, nutmeg and the other ingredients, put the lid on and cook on High for 2 hours.
2. Divide the oatmeal into bowls and serve for breakfast.

Nutrition: Calories 218, Fat 2.8g, Cholesterol 3mg, Sodium 65mg, Carbohydrate 36.7g, Fiber 4g, Sugars 10.4g, Protein 9g, Potassium 375mg

Breakfast Nuts and Squash Bowls

Preparation time: 10 minutes | Cooking time: 8 hours | Servings: 4

Ingredients:
- 1 teaspoon cinnamon powder
- ½ teaspoon nutmeg, ground
- ½ cup almonds
- ½ cup walnuts
- A splash of water
- 2 apples, peeled, cored and cubed
- 1 butternut squash, peeled and cubed
- 1 tablespoon stevia
- 1 cup coconut milk

Directions:
1. Put almonds and walnuts in your blender, add a splash of water, blend really well and transfer to your slow cooker.
2. Add apples, squash, cinnamon, stevia, nutmeg and coconut milk, stir, cover and cook on Low for 8 hours.
3. Stir, divide into bowls and serve.

Nutrition: Calories 392, Fat 29.8g, Cholesterol 0mg, Sodium 19mg, Carbohydrate 30.5g, Fiber 7g, Sugars 19.8g, Protein 8.2g, Potassium 517mg

Leeks, Kale and Sweet Potato Mix

Preparation time: 10 minutes | Cooking time: 6 hours and 10 minutes | Servings: 4

Ingredients:
- 2/3 cup sweet potato, grated
- 1 and 1/3 cups leek, chopped
- 2 tablespoons olive oil
- 8 eggs
- 1 cup kale, chopped
- 2 teaspoons garlic, minced
- 1 and ½ cups sausage, chopped

Directions:
1. Heat up a pan with the oil over medium-high heat; add sausage, stir, and brown for 2-3 minutes and transfer to your slow cooker.
2. Add garlic, sweet potatoes, kale and crack the eggs.
3. Stir, cover, cook on Low for 6 hours, divide between plates and serve.

Nutrition: Calories 279, Fat 17.8g, Cholesterol 336mg, Sodium 224mg, Carbohydrate 14g, Fiber 1.9g, Sugars 4g, Protein 14.8g, Potassium 447mg

Brown Rice and Plums

Preparation time: 10 minutes | Cooking time: 3 hours | Servings: 4

Ingredients:
- 1 cup brown rice
- 2 cups almond milk
- ½ cup plums, pitted and cubed

- 1 tablespoon maple syrup
- 1 teaspoon vanilla extract

Directions:
1. In your slow cooker, combine the rice with the milk and the other ingredients, put the lid on and cook on Low for 3 hours.
2. Divide into bowls and serve for breakfast.

Nutrition: Calories 468, Fat 29.9g, Cholesterol 0mg, Sodium 20mg, Carbohydrate 47.3g, Fiber 4.4g, Sugars 8g, Protein 6.4g, Potassium 468mg

Egg Casserole

Preparation time: 10 minutes | Cooking time: 8 hours and 10 minutes | Servings: 4

Ingredients:
- 2 garlic cloves, minced
- 1 tablespoon olive oil
- 1 red onion, chopped
- 3 sausage links, sliced
- Black pepper to the taste
- 1 red bell pepper, chopped
- 1 teaspoon dill, chopped
- 1 cup coconut milk
- 2 sweet potatoes, grated
- 12 eggs
- A pinch of red pepper, crushed

Directions:
1. Heat up a pan with the oil over medium-high heat, add garlic, bell pepper and onion, stir and cook for 5 minutes.
2. Add grated sweet potato, red pepper and black pepper, stir and cook for 2 minutes more.
3. Transfer half of this to your slow cooker and spread on the bottom.
4. In a bowl, mix eggs with coconut milk and whisk well.
5. Pour half of the eggs over the veggies, add sausage, add another veggie layer and top with the rest of the eggs.
6. Sprinkle dill all over, cover, cook on Low for 8 hours, slice and serve for breakfast.

Nutrition: Calories 506, Fat 36g, Cholesterol 498mg, Sodium 611mg, Carbohydrate 27.4g, Fiber 4.5g, Sugars 10.8g, Protein 21.4g, Potassium 722mg

Maple Apples

Preparation time: 10 minutes | Cooking time: 1 hour and 30 minutes | Servings: 4

Ingredients:
- ½ cup maple syrup
- 1 teaspoon cinnamon powder
- ¼ teaspoon nutmeg, ground
- 1 tablespoon lemon juice
- 1 tablespoon avocado oil
- ¼ cup figs
- 1 teaspoon stevia
- ¼ cup walnuts, chopped
- 1 teaspoon lemon zest, grated
- ½ teaspoon orange zest, grated
- ½ cup water
- 4 apples, cored and tops cut off

Directions:
1. In a bowl, mix maple syrup with figs, stevia, walnuts, lemon and orange zest, half of the cinnamon, nutmeg, lemon juice and the oil, whisk really well and stuff apples with this mix.
2. Add the water to your slow cooker, add the rest of the cinnamon, stir, add apples inside, cover and cook on High for 1 hour and 30 minutes.
3. Divide apples between plates and serve for breakfast.

Nutrition: Calories 305, Fat 5.7g, Cholesterol 0mg, Sodium 9mg, Carbohydrate 66.7g, Fiber 7.4g, Sugars 52.9g, Protein 3g, Potassium 463mg

Quinoa and Eggs Mix

Preparation time: 10 minutes | Cooking time: 2 hours | Servings: 4

Ingredients:
- 2 cups coconut milk
- 2 cup quinoa
- 8 eggs, whisked
- A pinch of black pepper
- 1 teaspoon turmeric powder
- 1 teaspoon chili powder
- 1 teaspoon rosemary, dried

Directions:
1. In your slow cooker, combine the milk with the quinoa, eggs and the other ingredients, put the lid on and cook on High for 2 hours.
2. Divide into bowls and serve for breakfast.

Nutrition: Calories 720, Fat 42.7g, Cholesterol 327mg, Sodium 153mg, Carbohydrate 62.8g, Fiber 9.1g, Sugars 4.8g, Protein 26g, Potassium 942mg

Apples and Sauce

Preparation time: 10 minutes | Cooking time: 4 hours | Servings: 4

Ingredients:
- 1 tablespoon lemon juice
- ¼ cup cane juice
- 1/3 cup avocado oil
- ½ teaspoon cinnamon powder
- 5 apples, cored, peeled and cubed
- 1 teaspoon vanilla extract

Directions:
1. In your slow cooker, mix coconut oil with

cane juice, lemon juice, cinnamon and vanilla and whisk well.
2. Add apple cubes, toss well, cover, cook on High for 4 hours, divide into bowls and serve for breakfast.

Nutrition: Calories 219, Fat 2.9g, Cholesterol 0mg, Sodium 34mg, Carbohydrate 48.8g, Fiber 7.6g, Sugars 38.3g, Protein 1g, Potassium 364mg

Sweet Potato and Sausage Pie

Preparation time: 10 minutes | Cooking time: 8 hours | Servings: 4

Ingredients:
- 8 eggs, whisked
- 1 sweet potato, shredded
- 1 yellow onion, chopped
- 2 teaspoons basil, dried
- 2 teaspoons coconut oil, melted
- 1 tablespoon garlic powder
- 2 red bell peppers, chopped
- 1 pound sausage, crumbled
- Black pepper to the taste

Directions:
1. Grease your slow cooker with the oil; add sweet potatoes, sausage, garlic powder, bell pepper, onion, basil, salt and pepper.
2. Add the eggs, toss, cover, cook on Low for 8 hours, divide between plates and serve.

Nutrition: Calories 625, Fat 44.9g, Cholesterol 423mg, Sodium 1266mg, Carbohydrate 19.4g, Fiber 2.7g, Sugars 9.5g, Protein 35.2g, Potassium 763mg

Eggs and Bacon Mix

Preparation time: 10 minutes | Cooking time: 2 hours and 30 minutes | Servings: 4

Ingredients:
- 8 eggs, whisked
- ½ cup low-sodium bacon, cooked and chopped
- ½ cup coconut cream
- 1 red bell pepper, chopped
- 2 spring onions, chopped
- ½ teaspoon chili powder
- A pinch of black pepper

Directions:
1. In the slow cooker, mix the eggs with the bacon, cream and the other ingredients, put the lid on and cook on High for 2 hours and 30 minutes.
2. Divide between plates and serve for breakfast.

Nutrition: Calories 373, Fat 28.9g, Cholesterol 355mg, Sodium 390mg, Carbohydrate 5.3g, Fiber 1.4g, Sugars 3.4g, Protein 21.g, Potassium 280mg

Pumpkin Butter

Preparation time: 10 minutes | Cooking time: 4 hours | Servings: 8

Ingredients:
- 2 teaspoon lemon juice
- 30 ounces pumpkin puree
- ½ cup apple cider
- 1 teaspoon ginger, grated
- 1 teaspoon cinnamon powder
- 1 cup coconut sugar
- 1 teaspoon vanilla extract
- ¼ teaspoon cloves, ground
- ¼ teaspoon allspice, ground
- 1 teaspoon nutmeg, ground

Directions:
1. In your slow cooker, mix pumpkin puree with apple cider, coconut sugar, vanilla extract, cinnamon, nutmeg, lemon juice, ginger, cloves and allspice, stir, cover and cook on Low for 4 hours.
2. Blend using an immersion blender and serve for breakfast.

Nutrition: Calories 60, Fat 0.5g, Cholesterol 0mg, Sodium 11mg, Carbohydrate 13.3g, Fiber 3.2g, Sugars 5.4g, Protein 1.4g, Potassium 245mg

Pineapple and Carrot Mix

Preparation time: 10 minutes | Cooking time: 6 hours | Servings: 10

Ingredients:
- 2 tablespoons stevia
- 1 cup raisins
- 6 cups water
- 2 tablespoons cinnamon powder
- 14 ounces carrots, shredded
- 8 ounces canned pineapple, crushed
- 23 ounces natural applesauce
- 1 tablespoon pumpkin pie spice

Directions:
1. In your slow cooker, mix carrots with applesauce, raisins, stevia, cinnamon, pineapple and pumpkin pie spice, stir, cover, cook on Low for 6 hours, divide into bowls and serve for breakfast.

Nutrition: Calories 110, Fat 0.2g, Cholesterol 0mg, Sodium 42mg, Carbohydrate 29.6g, Fiber 3g, Sugars 19.6g, Protein 0.9g, Potassium 265mg

Ginger and Spring Onions Eggs Mix

Preparation time: 10 minutes | Cooking time: 2 hours | Servings: 4

Ingredients:

- 1 cup coconut cream
- 8 eggs, whisked
- ½ cup spring onions, chopped
- A pinch of black pepper
- 1 teaspoon coriander, ground
- ½ teaspoon ginger, grated
- 1 teaspoon hot paprika

Directions:
1. In your slow cooker, combine the cream with the eggs, spring onions and the other ingredients, put the lid on and cook on High for 2 hours.
2. Divide into bowls and serve for breakfast.

Nutrition: Calories 270, Fat 23.1g, Cholesterol 327mg, Sodium 153mg, Carbohydrate 5.3g, Fiber 1.7g, Sugars 3.1g, Protein 12.7g, Potassium 314mg

Spinach Pie

Preparation time: 10 minutes | Cooking time: 4 hours | Servings: 4

Ingredients:
- 8 eggs
- A pinch of black pepper
- 10 ounces spinach
- 2 cups baby Bella mushrooms, chopped
- 1 red bell pepper, chopped
- 1 cup coconut cream
- ½ cup almond flour
- ¼ teaspoons baking soda
- 1 and ½ cups low-fat cheese, shredded
- 2 tablespoons chives, chopped
- Cooking spray

Directions:
1. In a bowl, combine the eggs with coconut cream, chives and pepper and whisk.
2. Add almond flour, baking soda, cheese, bell pepper, mushrooms and spinach, toss, transfer to your slow cooker greased with cooking spray, cover and cook on Low for 4 hours.
3. Slice, divide between plates and serve for breakfast.

Nutrition: Calories 469, Fat 31.4g, Cholesterol 331mg, Sodium 523mg, Carbohydrate 28.6g, Fiber 6g, Sugars 7g, Protein 22.4g, Potassium 940mg

Creamy Veggie Omelet

Preparation time: 10 minutes | Cooking time: 3 hours | Servings: 4

Ingredients:
- 1 tablespoon coconut milk
- ½ red bell pepper, chopped
- Cooking spray
- 6 eggs
- 1 cup low-fat cheese, shredded
- ½ green bell pepper, chopped
- 1 small yellow onion, chopped
- A pinch of salt and black pepper

Directions:
1. Grease your slow cooker with cooking spray and spread onion, red and green bell pepper on the bottom.
2. In a bowl, mix the eggs with pepper, cheese and milk, whisk well, pour into the slow cooker, cover, cook on High for 3 hours, divide between plates and serve for breakfast.

Nutrition: Calories 235, Fat 17.1g, Cholesterol 275mg, Sodium 313mg, Carbohydrate 5g, Fiber 0.9g, Sugars 3.1g, Protein 15.9g, Potassium 210mg

Sausage and Hash Browns

Preparation time: 10 minutes | Cooking time: 3 hours | Servings: 4

Ingredients:
- 1 pound hash browns
- 1 and ½ cups low-sodium sausage, sliced
- ¼ cup spring onions, chopped
- 1 cup cherry tomatoes, halved
- 1 cup low-sodium veggie stock
- 1 jalapeno, chopped
- A pinch of black pepper

Directions:
1. In the slow cooker, combine the hash browns with the sausage and the other ingredients, put the lid on and cook on High for 3 hours.
2. Divide into bowls and serve.

Nutrition: Calories 315, Fat 14.3g, Cholesterol 0mg, Sodium 489mg, Carbohydrate 43.3g, Fiber 4.4g, Sugars 4.3g, Protein 4g, Potassium 785mg

Salmon Omelet

Preparation time: 10 minutes | Cooking time: 3 hours and 40 minutes | Servings: 3

Ingredients:
- 4 eggs, whisked
- ½ teaspoon olive oil
- ½ cup cashews, soaked, drained
- ¼ cup green onions, chopped
- 1 tablespoon lemon juice
- A pinch black pepper
- 4 ounces smoked salmon, chopped
- 1 cup almond milk
- 1 teaspoon garlic powder

Directions:
1. In your blender, mix cashews with milk, garlic powder, lemon juice, green onions and pepper, blend really well and leave aside.
2. Drizzle the oil in your slow cooker, add eggs, whisk, cover and cook on Low for 3 hours.

3. Add salmon, toss, cover, cook on Low for 40 minutes more, divide between plates, drizzle green onions sauce all over and serve.

Nutrition: Calories 457, Fat 38g, Cholesterol 227mg, Sodium 856mg, Carbohydrate 13.8g, Fiber 2.8g, Sugars 4.8g, Protein 40g, Potassium 524mg

Chicken Omelet

Preparation time: 10 minutes | Cooking time: 3 hours | Servings: 2

Ingredients:
- 1-ounce rotisserie chicken, shredded
- 1 tomato, chopped
- 1 teaspoon mustard
- 1 tablespoon avocado mayonnaise
- 1 small avocado, pitted, peeled and chopped
- Black pepper to the taste
- 4 eggs, whisked

Directions:
1. In a bowl, mix the eggs with chicken, avocado, tomato, mayo and mustard, toss, transfer to your slow cooker, cover, cook on Low for 3 hours, divide between plates and serve.

Nutrition: Calories 475, Fat 38g, Cholesterol 348mg, Sodium 800mg, Carbohydrate 19.9g, Fiber 7.6g, Sugars 6.6g, Protein 17.6g, Potassium 690mg

Dash Diet Slow Cooker Main Dish Recipes

Chicken Tacos

Preparation time: 10 minutes | Cooking time: 6 hours and 30 minutes | Servings: 6

Ingredients:
- 3 tablespoons lime juice
- 1 and ½ pounds chicken breast halves, boneless and skinless
- 1 teaspoon lemon zest, grated
- 1 cup salsa
- 12 fat-free tortillas
- 1 tablespoon chili powder
- 1 cup corn
- Low-fat sour cream for serving
- Shredded lettuce for serving

Directions:
1. In a bowl, mix the limejuice with chili powder and lemon zest and whisk.
2. Put the chicken in your slow cooker, add lime mix, toss, cover and cook on Low for 6 hours.
3. Transfer chicken to a cutting board, shred using 2 forks and return to the pot.
4. Add salsa and corn, cover and cook on Low for 30 minutes more.
5. Divide this mix on each tortilla, also add sour cream and lettuce wrap and serve.

Nutrition: Calories 543, Fat 12g, Cholesterol 104mg, Sodium 1083mg, Carbohydrate 66.8g, Fiber 8.1g, Sugars 6.8g, Protein 43.7g, Potassium 590mg.

Coconut Turkey Mix

Preparation time: 10 minutes | Cooking time: 6 hours | Servings: 4

Ingredients:
- 2 pounds turkey breast, skinless, boneless and sliced
- 1 cup coconut cream
- 1 teaspoon turmeric powder
- 1 teaspoon curry powder
- 1 teaspoon ginger, ground
- A pinch of black pepper
- ½ cup yellow onion, chopped
- 2 tablespoons avocado oil
- 2 garlic cloves, minced
- 1 tablespoon chives, chopped

Directions:
1. In your slow cooker, combine the turkey slices with the cream, turmeric and the other ingredients, put the lid on and cook on Low for 6 hours.
2. Divide between plates and serve with a side salad.

Nutrition: Calories 397, Fat 19.1g, Cholesterol 98mg, Sodium 2313mg, Carbohydrate 16.1g, Fiber 3.5g, Sugars 10.7g, Protein 40.6g, Potassium 922mg

Quinoa Casserole

Preparation time: 10 minutes | Cooking time: 4 hours | Servings: 4

Ingredients:
- 1 cup low-fat Swiss cheese, shredded
- 12 ounces tomatillos, chopped
- 1 red bell pepper, chopped
- 1 pint cherry tomatoes, chopped
- ½ cup white onion, chopped
- 2 tablespoon
- oregano, chopped
- A pinch of black pepper
- 1 cup quinoa
- 1 tablespoon lime juice
- 2 pounds yellow summer squash, cubed
- Cooking spray

Directions:
1. In a bowl, mix the tomatoes with tomatillos, onion, lime juice and black pepper and toss.
2. Grease your slow cooker with the cooking spray and add quinoa.

3. Add half of the cheese and the squash and spread.
4. Add the rest of the cheese and the tomatillo mix, spread, cover and cook on Low for 4 hours.
5. Divide between plates, sprinkle oregano on top and serve.

Nutrition: Calories 388, Fat 11.1g, Cholesterol 25mg, Sodium 203mg, Carbohydrate 50.1g, Fiber 10.1g, Sugars 8.3g, Protein 21.1g, Potassium 800mg.

Quinoa Curry

Preparation time: 10 minutes | Cooking time: 4 hours | Servings: 6

Ingredients:
- 2 garlic cloves, minced
- 1 sweet potato, chopped
- 2 cups green beans, halved
- 1 tablespoon ginger, grated
- 1 teaspoon turmeric powder
- 2 teaspoons tamari sauce
- 1 carrot, chopped
- 1 small yellow onion, chopped
- 15 ounces canned chickpeas, drained and rinsed
- 28 ounces canned tomatoes, chopped
- 28 ounces coconut milk
- ¼ cup quinoa
- 1 and ½ cups water
- 1 teaspoon chili flakes

Directions:
1. In your slow cooker, combine the potato with green beans, carrot, onion, chickpeas, tomatoes, coconut milk, quinoa, garlic, ginger, turmeric, tamari, water and chili flakes, toss, cover and cook on Low for 4 hours.
2. Divide into bowls and serve.

Nutrition: Calories 657, Fat 36.7g, Cholesterol 0mg, Sodium 173mg, Carbohydrate 70.1g, Fiber 19.9g, Sugars 18.3g, Protein 20.5g, Potassium 1565mg.

Shrimp and Green Beans Mix

Preparation time: 10 minutes | Cooking time: 1 hour | Servings: 4

Ingredients:
- 2 pounds shrimp, peeled and deveined
- ½ pound green beans, trimmed and halved
- 1 tablespoon avocado oil
- ½ cup low-sodium veggie stock
- 1 tablespoon tomato juice
- ½ cup red onion, chopped
- 1 teaspoon hot paprika
- 2 tablespoons cilantro, chopped

Directions:
1. In the slow cooker, combine the shrimp with the green beans, oil and the other ingredients, put the lid on and cook on High for 1 hour.
2. Divide into bowls and serve.

Nutrition: Calories 301, Fat 4.4g, Cholesterol 478mg, Sodium 604mg, Carbohydrate 9.6g, Fiber 2.4g, Sugars 1.7g, Protein 53g, Potassium 546mg

Delicious Black Bean Chili

Preparation time: 10 minutes | Cooking time: 4 hours | Servings: 4

Ingredients:
- 2 garlic cloves, minced
- 1 teaspoon chipotle chili pepper, chopped
- 1 and ½ cups red bell pepper, chopped
- 1 tablespoon chili powder
- 1 cup yellow onion, chopped
- 1 and ½ cups mushrooms, sliced
- 1 tablespoon olive oil
- ½ teaspoon cumin, ground
- 1 cup tomatoes, chopped
- 16 ounces canned black beans, drained and rinsed
- 2 tablespoons cilantro, chopped

Directions:
1. In your slow cooker, combine the red bell peppers with onion, mushrooms, oil, chili powder, garlic, chili pepper, cumin, black beans and tomatoes, stir, cover and cook on High for 4 hours.
2. Divide into bowls, sprinkle cilantro on top and serve.

Nutrition: Calories 469, Fat 5.9g, Cholesterol 0mg, Sodium 36mg, Carbohydrate 81.8g, Fiber 20g, Sugars 7.7g, Protein 27g, Potassium 2047mg.

Chicken Stew

Preparation time: 10 minutes | Cooking time: 6 hours | Servings: 4

Ingredients:
- 2 pounds chicken breast, skinless, boneless and cubed
- 1 red onion, sliced
- 2 garlic cloves, minced
- 1 cup low-sodium chicken stock
- 1 teaspoon sweet paprika
- 1 teaspoon hot paprika
- 1 carrot, sliced
- 1 zucchini, cubed
- 2 tablespoons chives, chopped
- ½ cup tomato juice

Directions:
1. In your slow cooker, combine the chicken

with the onion, garlic and the other ingredients, put the lid on and cook on Low for 6 hours.
2. Stir the stew once more, divide into bowls and serve.

Nutrition: Calories 298, Fat 5.9g, Cholesterol 145mg, Sodium 251mg, Carbohydrate 8.3g, Fiber 1.9g, Sugars 4g, Protein 50.1g, Potassium 1149mg

Chicken and Veggies

Preparation time: 10 minutes | Cooking time: 4 hours | Servings: 4

Ingredients:
- 4 cups red potatoes, cubed
- 2 pounds chicken breasts, skinless and boneless
- 1 teaspoon oregano, dried
- 1 teaspoon cilantro, dried
- 2 garlic cloves, minced
- A pinch of black pepper
- ½ pounds green beans, trimmed
- ¼ cup olive oil
- 1/3 cup lemon juice
- ¼ teaspoon onion powder

Directions:
1. Put the chicken breasts in your slow cooker and add green beans and potatoes on top.
2. In a bowl, mix lemon juice with oil, cilantro, black pepper, oregano, and garlic and onion powder and whisk well.
3. Pour this into the slow cooker, cover and cook on High for 4 hours.
4. Divide chicken and veggies between plates and serve.

Nutrition: Calories 670, Fat 29.9g, Cholesterol 202mg, Sodium 212mg, Carbohydrate 29.2g, Fiber 4.8g, Sugars 2.8g, Protein 69.8g, Potassium 1392mg.

Succulent Beef Roast

Preparation time: 10 minutes | Cooking time: 8 hours | Servings: 8

Ingredients:
- 1 tablespoon sage, dried
- ¼ cup balsamic vinegar
- 1/3 cup low sodium veggie stock
- ½ teaspoon garlic powder
- 2 pounds roast beef
- 1 tablespoon cider vinegar
- 1 tablespoon stevia

Directions:
1. Put the roast in your slow cooker and pour the stock over it.
2. In a bowl, mix sage with garlic powder, vinegar, cider vinegar and stevia, whisk well, pour into the slow cooker as well, cover and cook on Low for 8 hours.
3. Shred the meat, divide it between plates, drizzle cooking juices all over and serve.

Nutrition: Calories 215, Fat 7.1g, Cholesterol 101mg, Sodium 81mg, Carbohydrate 1.4g, Fiber 0.1g, Sugars 0.1g, Protein 34.5g, Potassium 467mg

Chicken and Peppers Soup

Preparation time: 10 minutes | Cooking time: 6 hours | Servings: 4

Ingredients:
- 2 teaspoons olive oil
- 2 pounds chicken breast, skinless, boneless, cubed and browned
- 1 red bell pepper, chopped
- 1 green bell pepper, chopped
- 1 orange bell pepper, chopped
- 1 red onion, chopped
- 1 carrot, sliced
- 6 cups low-sodium chicken stock
- ½ cup red enchilada sauce, low-sodium
- 1 teaspoon chili powder
- 1 tablespoon parsley, chopped

Directions:
1. In the slow cooker, combine the chicken with the peppers and the other ingredients, put the lid on and cook on Low for 6 hours.
2. Divide into bowls and serve.

Nutrition: Calories 33, Fat 8.8g, Cholesterol 145mg, Sodium 536mg, Carbohydrate 11.3g, Fiber 3.6g, Sugars 6.2g, Protein 51.1g, Potassium 1054mg

Turkey Chili

Preparation time: 10 minutes | Cooking time: 8 hours | Servings: 6

Ingredients:
- 28 ounces canned tomatoes, no-salt-added, crushed
- 2 tablespoons chili powder
- 2 tablespoons sweet paprika
- 1 tablespoon garlic powder
- 1 pound turkey meat, ground
- 15 ounces canned black beans, no-salt-added, drained and rinsed
- 15 ounces canned kidney beans, no-salt-added, drained and rinsed
- 3 tablespoons onion powder
- ¼ cup cumin, ground
- 1 red bell pepper, chopped
- 1 green bell pepper, chopped
- 2 tablespoons oregano, chopped
- 1 oz jalapeno pepper
- 1 garlic clove, minced
- 1 yellow onion, chopped
- 1 and ½ cup corn
- 9 ounces tomato sauce, no-salt-added

Directions:
1. In a bowl, mix chili powder with garlic powder, onion powder, cumin, oregano, paprika and jalapeno and whisk well.
2. Put the meat in your slow cooker, add spice mix and toss well.
3. Also, add garlic, onion, corn, red and green bell pepper, tomatoes, kidney beans, black beans and tomato sauce, toss, cover and cook on Low for 8 hours.
4. Divide into bowls and serve.

Nutrition: Calories 747, Fat 8.3g, Cholesterol 57mg, Sodium 337mg, Carbohydrate 116.7g, Fiber 29.1g, Sugars 14.1g, Protein 59.2g, Potassium 3159mg

Creamy Beef Mix

Preparation time: 10 minutes | Cooking time: 8 hours | Servings: 4

Ingredients:
- 1 tablespoon avocado oil
- 2 pounds beef stew meat, cubed and browned
- 4 spring onions, chopped
- 1 cup coconut cream
- ½ cup low-sodium veggie stock
- A pinch of black pepper
- 4 garlic cloves, minced
- 1 teaspoon nutmeg, ground
- 1 tablespoon chives, chopped
- 1 tablespoon basil, chopped

Directions:
1. In the slow cooker, combine the beef with the oil, spring onions and the other ingredients, put the lid on and cook on Low for 8 hours.
2. Toss the mix again, divide into bowls and serve.

Nutrition: Calories 578, Fat 29.1g, Cholesterol 203mg, Sodium 210mg, Carbohydrate 6.5g, Fiber 2.1g, Sugars 2.7g, Protein 70.7g, Potassium 1142mg

Pulled Chicken

Preparation time: 10 minutes | Cooking time: 5 hours | Servings: 4

Ingredients:
- 8 ounces tomato sauce, no-salt-added
- 4 ounces canned green chilies, drained and chopped
- 3 tablespoons cider vinegar
- 1 teaspoon chipotle chili, dried and ground
- 1 yellow onion, chopped
- 2 tablespoons stevia
- 1 tablespoon cider vinegar
- 2 teaspoons dried mustard
- 1 tablespoon sweet paprika
- 1 garlic clove, minced
- 1 tablespoon tomato paste
- 2 and ½ pounds chicken thighs, boneless and skinless

Directions:
1. In a bowl, mix the tomato sauce with green chilies, stevia, vinegar, paprika, tomato paste, cider vinegar, dried mustard and chipotle chili and whisk really well.
2. Pour this into your slow cooker, add chicken thighs, onion and garlic, toss, cover and cook on Low for 5 hours.
3. Shred the meat using 2 forks, divide everything between plates and serve.

Nutrition: Calories 677, Fat 23.6g, Cholesterol 252mg, Sodium 578mg, Carbohydrate 35.8g, Fiber 10.7g, Sugars 16.2g, Protein 87g, Potassium 1550mg.

Lime Chicken Mix

Preparation time: 10 minutes | Cooking time: 5 hours | Servings: 4

Ingredients:
- 1 pound chicken breasts, skinless, boneless and cubed
- Juice of 1 lime
- Zest of 1 lime, grated
- 1 teaspoon coriander, ground
- 1 teaspoon rosemary, dried
- 1 cup fat-free yogurt
- 1 tablespoon chives, chopped
- A pinch of black pepper
- 2 garlic cloves, minced
- 1 cup coconut cream

Directions:
1. In the slow cooker, combine the chicken with the lime juice, lime zest and the other ingredients, toss, cover and cook on Low for 5 hours.
2. Divide everything into bowls and serve.

Nutrition: Calories 396, Fat 22.9g, Cholesterol 102mg, Sodium 155mg, Carbohydrate 10.5g, Fiber 2g, Sugars 7g, Protein 37.9g, Potassium 619mg

Mediterranean Chicken

Preparation time: 10 minutes | Cooking time: 2 hours and 30 minutes | Servings: 4

Ingredients:
- Black pepper to the taste
- 2 tablespoons scallions, chopped
- 1 pound chicken breasts, skinless and boneless
- 2 tomatoes, chopped
- 1 cup low-sodium chicken stock
- ¾ cup whole wheat orzo
- ½ cup black olives, pitted
- ½ red bell pepper, chopped

- 1 yellow onion, sliced
- Zest of 1 lemon,
- grated
- Juice of 1 lemon

Directions:
1. In your slow cooker, mix chicken with tomatoes, stock, bell pepper, onion, lemon zest, lemon juice and black pepper to the taste, cover and cook on High for 2 hours.
2. Add black olives and orzo, toss, cover, cook on high for 30 minutes more, divide everything between plates and serve with chopped scallions on top.

Nutrition: Calories 334, Fat 12.1g, Cholesterol 101mg, Sodium 563mg, Carbohydrate 20.5g, Fiber 3.1g, Sugars 6.2g, Protein 35.8g, Potassium 519mg.

Chicken and Mushroom Soup

Preparation time: 10 minutes | Cooking time: 6 hours | Servings: 4

Ingredients:
- 1 tablespoon olive oil
- 1 pound chicken thighs, boneless, skinless, cubed and browned
- ½ pound white mushrooms, sliced
- 1 yellow onion, chopped
- 6 cups low-sodium chicken stock
- A pinch of black pepper
- 1 teaspoon ginger, grated
- 1 carrot, chopped
- 1 cup baby spinach
- 1 tablespoon parsley, chopped

Directions:
1. In the slow cooker, combine the chicken with the mushrooms, oil and the other ingredients, put the lid on and cook on Low for 6 hours.
2. Divide into bowls and serve.

Nutrition: Calories 286, Fat 12.2g, Cholesterol 101mg, Sodium 321mg, Carbohydrate 6.6g, Fiber 1.8g, Sugars 3g, Protein 36.8g, Potassium 598mg

Delicious Veggie Soup

Preparation time: 10 minutes | Cooking time: 9 hours and 30 minutes | Servings: 6

Ingredients:
- 15 ounces canned kidney beans, no-salt-added, drained and rinsed
- 14 ounces low-sodium chicken stock
- ¼ cup parsley, chopped
- 2 teaspoons oregano, dried
- Black pepper to the taste
- ½ cup pearl barley
- ½ cup corn
- 14 ounces canned tomatoes, no-salt-added and drained
- 3 cups fat-free milk
- 1 cup mushrooms, sliced
- 1 carrot, sliced
- 1 cup yellow onion, chopped
- 1 celery stalk, chopped
- 3 garlic cloves, minced
- ½ cup peas
- ½ cup green beans

Directions:
1. In your slow cooker, mix the kidney beans with barley, corn, tomatoes, mushrooms, carrot, onion, celery, garlic, peas, green beans, oregano, black pepper and stock, stir, cover and cook on Low for 9 hours.
2. Add milk and parsley, stir, cover, cook on Low for 30 minutes more, ladle into bowls and serve.

Nutrition: Calories 421, Fat 2.4g, Cholesterol 2mg, Sodium 318mg, Carbohydrate 79.6g, Fiber 16.7g, Sugars 13.7g, Protein 24.8g, Potassium 1573mg.

Turkey and Tomatoes

Preparation time: 10 minutes | Cooking time: 6 hours | Servings: 4

Ingredients:
- 2 tablespoons olive oil
- 2 pounds turkey breast, skinless, boneless and cut into strips
- 2 cups cherry tomatoes, halved
- 2 tablespoons tomato juice
- 1 cup veggie stock, low-sodium
- 1 red chili pepper, minced
- ½ teaspoon red pepper flakes, crushed
- 1 teaspoon rosemary, dried
- 1 tablespoon lime juice
- 1 tablespoon cilantro, chopped

Directions:
1. In the slow cooker, combine the turkey with the tomatoes, tomato juice and the other ingredients, put the lid on and cook on Low for 6 hours..
2. Divide everything between plates and serve.

Nutrition: Calories 320, Fat 11g, Cholesterol 98mg, Sodium 2362mg, Carbohydrate 14.5g, Fiber 2.5g, Sugars 11g, Protein 39.6g, Potassium 929mg

Chicken and Rice Soup

Preparation time: 10 minutes | Cooking time: 8 hours and 30 minutes | Servings: 4

Ingredients:
- 2 yellow onions, chopped
- 3 carrots, chopped
- 8 ounces corn
- 1 tablespoon olive oil
- 1 tablespoon salt-free tomato paste
- ½ teaspoon thyme, dried
- 4 garlic clove, minced
- 8 cups low-sodium chicken stock
- 2 celery ribs, sliced
- 2 bay leaves

- 2 pounds chicken thighs, skinless and boneless
- 2 tablespoons water
- 1 tablespoon jalapeno pepper powder
- 1 cup wild rice
- 2 tablespoons cornstarch
- 2 tablespoon parsley, chopped

Directions:

1. In your slow cooker, mix the onions with garlic, oil, tomato paste, thyme, stock, carrots, corn, celery, bay leaves and chicken thighs, cover and cook on Low for 8 hours.
2. Add cornstarch mixed with water, jalapeno and rice, stir, cover and cook on Low for 30 minutes more.
3. Ladle soup into bowls, discard bay leaves, sprinkle parsley on top and serve.

Nutrition: Calories 958, Fat 24.7g, Cholesterol 202mg, Sodium 569mg, Carbohydrate 106.1g, Fiber 14.9g, Sugars 16.3g, Protein 85.4g, Potassium 1902mg.

Delicious Black Bean Soup

Preparation time: 10 minutes | Cooking time: 8 hours and 5 minutes | Servings: 4

Ingredients:

- 1 tablespoon olive oil
- 50 ounces canned black beans, no-salt-added, drained and rinsed
- 1 yellow onion, chopped
- 4 cups water
- 4 garlic cloves, minced
- A pinch of black pepper
- 4 cups low-sodium veggie stock
- 1 yellow bell pepper, chopped
- 1 red bell pepper, chopped
- 1 teaspoon cumin, ground
- ½ cup cilantro, chopped
- Juice of 2 limes

Directions:

1. Heat up a pan with the oil over medium-high heat, add onion and garlic, stir and cook for 2 minutes.
2. Add yellow and red bell pepper, stir, cook for 3 minutes more and transfer everything to your slow cooker.
3. Add beans, cumin, water, stock and black pepper, stir, cover and cook on Low for 8 minutes.
4. Add cilantro and lime juice, stir, ladle into bowls and serve.

Nutrition: Calories 1291, Fat 8.8g, Cholesterol 0mg, Sodium 213mg, Carbohydrate 232.1g, Fiber 55.4g, Sugars 12.4g, Protein 77.7g, Potassium 5442mg.

Ginger Beef Mix

Preparation time: 10 minutes | Cooking time: 6 hours | Servings: 4

Ingredients:

- 1 pound beef stew meat, cut into strips and browned
- 2 tablespoons ginger
- ¾ cup low-sodium beef stock
- 1 red onion, chopped
- ½ cup coconut cream
- 1 tablespoon olive oil
- 2 tablespoons coconut aminos
- 1 tablespoon oregano, chopped
- 1 tablespoon rosemary, chopped

Directions:

1. In the slow cooker, mix the beef with the ginger, stock and the other ingredients, put the lid on and cook on Low for 6 hours.
2. Divide everything between plates and serve right away.

Nutrition: Calories 346, Fat 18.2g, Cholesterol 101mg, Sodium 116mg, Carbohydrate 8.9g, Fiber 2.4g, Sugars 2.3g, Protein 36.2g, Potassium 639mg

Beet Soup

Preparation time: 10 minutes | Cooking time: 7 hours | Servings: 6

Ingredients:

- 1 and ¼ pounds beets, peeled and cut into wedges
- 4 and ½ cups low-sodium veggie stock
- 2 tablespoons apple cider vinegar
- 1 tablespoon stevia
- 2 tablespoons olive oil
- 1 red onion, chopped
- 2 garlic cloves, minced
- 1 apple, peeled, cored and sliced
- A pinch of black pepper

Directions:

1. Heat up a pan with the oil over medium-high heat, add the onion and the garlic stir, cook for 2-3 minutes and transfer to your slow cooker.
2. Add beets, apple, stock, vinegar, stevia and black pepper, cover and cook on Low for 7 hours.
3. Puree the soup using an immersion blender, ladle soup into bowls and serve.

Nutrition: Calories 122, Fat 4.9g, Cholesterol 0mg, Sodium 179mg, Carbohydrate 19.5g, Fiber 3.2g, Sugars 13g, Protein 2g, Potassium 363mg.

Tarragon Chicken and Corn

Preparation time: 10 minutes | Cooking time: 5 hours | Servings: 4

Ingredients:

- 2 pounds chicken breast, skinless, boneless and cubed
- 1 and ½ cups corn
- 1 cup chicken stock, low-sodium
- 1 tablespoon tarragon, chopped
- 1 cup coconut cream
- 2 celery sticks, chopped
- 3 garlic cloves, minced
- A pinch of black pepper

Directions:

1. In your slow cooker, combine the chicken with the corn, stock and the other ingredients, put the lid on and cook on Low for 5 hours.
2. Divide the mix between plates and serve.

Nutrition: Calories 455, Fat 20.7g, Cholesterol 145mg, Sodium 184mg, Carbohydrate 15.8g, Fiber 3.3g, Sugars 4.2g, Protein 52g, Potassium 1228mg

Delicious Tomato Cream

Preparation time: 10 minutes | Cooking time: 4 hours | Servings: 8

Ingredients:

- 56 ounces tomatoes, chopped
- 4 tablespoon non-fat butter
- 1 teaspoon oregano, dried
- 1 bay leaf
- 1 small yellow onion, chopped
- 2 cups low-sodium veggie stock
- ½ teaspoon garlic powder
- A pinch of black pepper
- 1 teaspoon thyme, dried
- 1 cup fat-free milk

Directions:

1. In your slow cooker, combine the tomatoes with the onion, stock, thyme, oregano, garlic powder, black pepper, bay leaf, butter and milk, stir, cover and cook on High for 4 hours.
2. Discard the bay leaf, puree the soup in batches in your blender, ladle into bowls and serve.

Nutrition: Calories 71, Fat 0.6g, Cholesterol 1mg, Sodium 94mg, Carbohydrate 14.1g, Fiber 2.9g, Sugars 7.5g, Protein 3.3g, Potassium 538mg

Shrimp and Rice

Preparation time: 10 minutes | Cooking time: 2 hours and 30 minutes | Servings: 4

Ingredients:

- 1 red onion, chopped
- 1 pound shrimp, peeled and deveined
- 1 cup wild rice
- 2 teaspoons avocado oil
- 2 cups low-sodium chicken stock
- 1 teaspoon sweet paprika
- 1 teaspoon coriander, ground
- A pinch of black pepper
- 1 teaspoon hot sauce
- 1 tablespoon chives, chopped

Directions:

1. In your slow cooker, combine the rice with the stock, onion and the other ingredients except the shrimp, put the lid on and cook on High for 2 hours.
2. Add the shrimp, cook the mix for 30 minutes more on High, divide everything between plates and serve.

Nutrition: Calories 301, Fat 2.8g, Cholesterol 239mg, Sodium 348mg, Carbohydrate 35.3g, Fiber 3.4g, Sugars 2.3g, Protein 33.2g, Potassium 428mg

Rich Lentils Soup

Preparation time: 10 minutes | Cooking time: 6 hours | Servings: 6

Ingredients:

- 4 cups red lentils
- 1 yellow onion, chopped
- 6 carrots, chopped
- Zest of 1 lemon, grated
- Juice of 1 lemon
- 4 garlic cloves, minced
- 1 yellow bell pepper, chopped
- A pinch of cayenne pepper
- 4 cups low sodium chicken stock
- 4 cups water
- 1 tablespoon rosemary, chopped

Directions:

1. In your slow cooker, mix the onion with the carrots, garlic, bell pepper, cayenne, lentils, stock and water, stir, cover and cook on Low for 6 hours.
2. Add lemon zest, lemon juice and rosemary, stir, ladle into bowls and serve.

Nutrition: Calories 509, Fat 1.6g, Cholesterol 1mg, Sodium 103mg, Carbohydrate 89g, Fiber 42g, Sugars 7.7g, Protein 35.6g, Potassium 1514mg

Broccoli and Cauliflower Soup

Preparation time: 10 minutes | Cooking time: 8 hours | Servings: 4

Ingredients:

- 3 cups broccoli florets
- A pinch of black pepper
- 1 cup fat-free milk
- 2 cups cauliflower florets
- 6 ounce low-fat cheddar cheese, shredded
- 2 garlic cloves, minced
- ½ cup shallots, chopped
- 1 carrot, chopped
- 3 and ½ cups low sodium veggie stock
- 1 cup non-fat Greek yogurt

Directions:
1. In your slow cooker, mix the broccoli with cauliflower, garlic, shallots, carrot, stock and black pepper, cover and cook on Low for 8 hours.
2. Transfer the soup to a blender, add milk and cheese and pulse well.
3. Add the yogurt, pulse again, ladle into bowls and serve.

Nutrition: Calories 303, Fat 14.4g, Cholesterol 46mg, Sodium 486mg, Carbohydrate 22.9g, Fiber 3.4g, Sugars 12.2g, Protein 20.2g, Potassium 626mg

Pork Chops and Sprouts

Preparation time: 10 minutes | Cooking time: 6 hours | Servings: 4

Ingredients:
- 2 pounds pork chops
- ½ pound Brussels sprouts, trimmed and halved
- 1 cup tomato juice
- ½ teaspoon coriander, ground
- ½ teaspoon rosemary, dried
- 3 garlic cloves, minced
- ½ tablespoon chives, chopped
- A pinch of black pepper

Directions:
1. In your slow cooker, combine the pork chops with the sprouts, tomato juice and the other ingredients, put the lid on and cook on Low for 6 hours.
2. Divide the mix between plates and serve.

Nutrition: Calories 765, Fat 56.6g, Cholesterol 195mg, Sodium 337mg, Carbohydrate 8.6g, Fiber 2.5g, Sugars 3.4g, Protein 53.3g, Potassium 1152mg

Butternut Squash Cream

Preparation time: 10 minutes | Cooking time: 4 hours | Servings: 6

Ingredients:
- 1 yellow onion, chopped
- 1 sage spring
- 2 cups low sodium veggie stock
- 2 garlic cloves, minced
- 1 carrot, sliced
- 1 green apple, cored, peeled and chopped
- 1 medium butternut squash, peeled, deseeded and chopped
- A pinch of cinnamon powder
- A pinch of nutmeg, ground
- A pinch of black pepper
- A pinch of cayenne pepper
- ½ cup coconut milk

Directions:
1. In your slow cooker, mix the stock with garlic, carrot, apple, squash, onion, sage, black pepper, cayenne, nutmeg and cinnamon, cover and cook on High for 4 hours.
2. Add coconut milk, discard sage, blend the soup using an immersion blender, ladle into bowls and serve.

Nutrition: Calories 94, Fat 4.9g, Cholesterol 0mg, Sodium 59mg, Carbohydrate 12.7g, Fiber 2.5g, Sugars 6.7g, Protein 1.1g, Potassium 241mg

Chickpeas Mix

Preparation time: 10 minutes | Cooking time: 4 hours and 5 minutes | Servings: 6

Ingredients:
- 1 yellow onion, chopped
- 2 red Thai chilies, chopped
- ½ teaspoon turmeric powder
- 1 tablespoon ginger, grated
- 1 tablespoon olive oil
- 4 garlic cloves, minced
- 4 ounces no-salt-added tomato paste
- 2 cups low sodium veggie stock
- 6 ounces canned chickpeas, drained and rinsed
- A pinch of black pepper
- 2 tablespoons garam masala
- 2 tablespoons parsley, chopped

Directions:
1. Heat up a pan with the oil over medium-high heat, add ginger, onions, garlic, pepper, Thai chilies, garam masala and turmeric, stir, cook for 5-6 minutes more and transfer everything to your slow cooker.
2. Add stock, chickpeas and tomato paste, stir, cover and cook on Low for 4 hours.
3. Add parsley, stir, divide into bowls and serve.

Nutrition: Calories 163, Fat 4.2g, Cholesterol 0mg, Sodium 84mg, Carbohydrate 25.2g, Fiber 6.1g, Sugars 6.6g, Protein 7.1g, Potassium 307mg

Red Beans and Chicken Mix

Preparation time: 10 minutes | Cooking time: 6 hours | Servings: 4

Ingredients:
- 1 pound chicken breast, skinless, boneless, cubed and browned
- 1 cup canned red kidney beans, no-salt-added, drained and rinsed
- 1 teaspoon rosemary, ground
- 1 cup cherry tomatoes, halved
- 2 teaspoons olive oil
- 1 red onion, chopped
- 1 cup low-sodium chicken stock
- A pinch of black pepper
- 1 tablespoon cilantro,

chopped

Directions:
1. In the slow cooker, combine the chicken with the beans, rosemary and the other ingredients, put the lid on and cook on Low for 6 hours.
2. Divide into bowls and serve.

Nutrition: Calories 221, Fat 5.6g, Cholesterol 73mg, Sodium 115mg, Carbohydrate 15g, Fiber 4.8g, Sugars 3.4g, Protein 28.5g, Potassium 786mg

Navy Beans Stew

Preparation time: 10 minutes | Cooking time: 12 hours | Servings: 6

Ingredients:
- 4 tablespoons stevia
- 1 cup water
- 1 pound navy beans, soaked overnight and drained
- 1 cup maple syrup
- 1 cup no-salt tomato sauce
- ¼ cup no-salt-added tomato paste
- ¼ cup olive oil
- ¼ cup apple cider vinegar
- ¼ cup mustard

Directions:
1. In your slow cooker, mix beans with maple syrup, tomato sauce, stevia, water, tomato paste, mustard, oil and vinegar, stir, cover, cook on Low for 12 hours, divide into bowls and serve.

Nutrition: Calories 509, Fat 11.6g, Cholesterol 0mg, Sodium 25mg, Carbohydrate 89.8g, Fiber 20g, Sugars 36.5g, Protein 19.1g, Potassium 1195mg

Potatoes Stew

Preparation time: 10 minutes | Cooking time: 3 hours | Servings: 4

Ingredients:
- 1 pound gold potatoes, peeled and cubed
- 1 pound spinach, torn
- 1 small onion, chopped
- 2 tablespoons water
- 1 tablespoon olive oil
- ½ teaspoon garam masala
- ½ teaspoon chili powder
- ½ teaspoon cumin, ground
- ½ teaspoon coriander, ground
- Black pepper to the taste

Directions:
1. In your slow cooker, mix potatoes with onion, water, oil, cumin, coriander, garam masala, chili, spinach and black pepper, stir, cover, cook on High for 3 hours, divide into bowls and serve.

Nutrition: Calories 173, Fat 5.6g, Cholesterol 0mg, Sodium 375mg, Carbohydrate 28.4g, Fiber 6.2g, Sugars 5g, Protein 5.3g, Potassium 1183mg

Broccoli Soup

Preparation time: 10 minutes | Cooking time: 3 hours | Servings: 4

Ingredients:
- 1 yellow onion, chopped
- 1 pound broccoli florets
- 2 teaspoons olive oil
- 5 cups low-sodium veggie stock
- 1 cup coconut cream
- 1 teaspoon rosemary, dried
- 3 garlic cloves, minced
- 1 teaspoon thyme, dried

Directions:
1. In the instant pot, combine the broccoli with the onion, stock and the other ingredients except the cream, put the lid on and cook on High for 3 hours.
2. Add the cream, blend the soup using an immersion blender, divide into bowls and serve.

Nutrition: Calories 231, Fat 17.1g, Cholesterol 0mg, Sodium 136mg, Carbohydrate 15.8g, Fiber 5.1g, Sugars 5.1g, Protein 7.5g, Potassium 571mg

Easy Navy Beans Soup

Preparation time: 10 minutes | Cooking time: 4 hours | Servings: 6

Ingredients:
- 1 pounds navy beans, dried
- 2 gold potatoes, cubed
- 1 pound carrots, sliced
- 1 yellow onion, chopped
- 2 quarts low-sodium veggie stock
- 2 teaspoons dill, chopped
- Black pepper to the taste
- 1 cup sun-dried tomatoes, chopped
- 4 tablespoons parsley, chopped

Directions:
1. In your slow cooker, mix beans with onion, stock, pepper, potatoes, carrots, tomatoes, dill and parsley, stir, cover, cook on High for 4 hours, ladle into bowls and serve.

Nutrition: Calories 359, Fat 2.2g, Cholesterol 0mg, Sodium 434mg, Carbohydrate 66.1g, Fiber 21.9g, Sugars 11.4g, Protein 18.6g, Potassium 1364mg

Turkey Soup

Preparation time: 10 minutes | Cooking time: 5 hours | Servings: 4

Ingredients:

- 1 pound turkey breast, skinless, boneless and cubed
- 1 yellow onion, chopped
- 1 teaspoon olive oil
- A pinch of black pepper
- 1 cup gold potatoes, peeled and cubed
- 1 fennel bulbs, sliced
- 1 cup celery, chopped
- 6 garlic cloves, minced
- 6 cups veggie stock, low-sodium
- ½ teaspoon coriander, ground
- 1 teaspoon chili powder
- 1 tablespoon parsley, chopped

Directions:
1. In the slow cooker, combine the turkey with the onion, oil, potatoes and the other ingredients, put the lid on and cook on Low for 5 hours.
2. Ladle the soup into bowls and serve.

Nutrition: Calories 218, Fat 3.4g, Cholesterol 49mg, Sodium 1421mg, Carbohydrate 23.3g, Fiber 4.7g, Sugars 7.6g, Protein 21.5g, Potassium 882mg

Black Beans and Mango Mix

Preparation time: 10 minutes | Cooking time: 6 hours and 15 minutes | Servings: 6

Ingredients:
- 2 mangoes, peeled, cored and chopped
- 1 yellow onion, chopped
- 1 tablespoon olive oil
- 1 red bell pepper, chopped
- 1 jalapeno, chopped
- 2 garlic cloves, minced
- 1 teaspoon ginger, grated
- 30 ounces canned black beans, no-salt-added, drained and rinsed
- ½ teaspoon stevia
- ½ teaspoon cumin, ground
- ½ teaspoon allspice, ground
- ½ teaspoon oregano, dried
- A pinch of black pepper
- 2 cups brown rice, cooked

Directions:
1. Heat up a pan with the oil over medium-high heat, add onion, garlic, ginger and jalapeno, stir, cook for 3 minutes and transfer to your slow cooker.
2. Add red bell pepper, cumin, allspice, oregano, black beans, stevia, water and pepper, stir, cover and cook on Low for 6 hours.
3. Add rice and mangoes, stir, cover, cook on Low for 10 minutes more, divide between plates and serve.

Nutrition: Calories 818, Fat 6.6g, Cholesterol 0mg, Sodium 13mg, Carbohydrate 157.6g, Fiber 26.4g, Sugars 20.2g, Protein 36.9g, Potassium 2544mg

Spinach Soup

Preparation time: 10 minutes | Cooking time: 10 hours | Servings: 8

Ingredients:
- 28 ounces canned tomatoes, no-salt-added and chopped
- 2 bay leaves
- 10 ounces baby spinach
- 4 cups veggie stock
- 2 celery ribs, chopped
- 2 carrots, chopped
- 1 garlic clove, minced
- 1 tablespoon cilantro, chopped
- 1 yellow onion, chopped
- 1 teaspoon oregano, dried
- ½ teaspoon red pepper flakes, crushed

Directions:
1. In your slow cooker, mix spinach with celery, carrots, garlic, onion, stock, tomatoes, bay leaves, oregano, cilantro, red pepper flakes, stir, cover, cook on Low for 10 hours, ladle into bowls and serve.

Nutrition: Calories 50, Fat 0.5g, Cholesterol 0mg, Sodium 317mg, Carbohydrate 10.4g, Fiber 3.5g, Sugars 5.2g, Protein 2.3g, Potassium 538mg

Shrimp and Quinoa Mix

Preparation time: 10 minutes | Cooking time: 2 hours | Servings: 4

Ingredients:
- 1 cup quinoa
- 2 cups low-sodium chicken stock
- 1 pound shrimp, peeled and deveined
- ½ teaspoon cumin, ground
- ½ teaspoon rosemary, dried
- A pinch of cayenne pepper
- 2 teaspoons sweet paprika
- Black pepper to the taste
- Juice of 1 lime
- ½ tablespoon olive oil
- 1 tablespoon chives, chopped

Directions:
1. In your slow cooker, combine the quinoa with the stock, shrimp and the other ingredients, put the lid on and cook on High for 2 hours.
2. Divide into bowls and serve.

Nutrition: Calories 354, Fat 8g, Cholesterol 239mg, Sodium 595mg, Carbohydrate 35.5g, Fiber 3.7g, Sugars 2.6g, Protein 33.4g, Potassium 478mg

Asian Salmon

Preparation time: 10 minutes | Cooking time: 3 hours | Servings: 2

Ingredients:
- 2 tablespoons maple syrup
- 2 medium salmon fillets, boneless
- Black pepper to the taste
- 2 tablespoons lemon juice
- 1 teaspoon sesame seeds
- 2 tablespoons low sodium soy sauce
- 16 ounces mixed broccoli and cauliflower florets

Directions:
1. Put the cauliflower and broccoli florets in your slow cooker and top with the salmon.
2. In a bowl, mix maple syrup with soy sauce and lemon juice, whisk, and pour over the salmon mix, season with black pepper to the taste, sprinkle sesame seeds on top and cook on Low for 3 hours.
3. Divide everything between plates and serve.

Nutrition: Calories 364, Fat 10.9g, Cholesterol 50mg, Sodium 1215mg, Carbohydrate 28.7g, Fiber 5.2g, Sugars 17g, Protein 32.9g, Potassium 535mg

Seafood Stew

Preparation time: 10 minutes | Cooking time: 3 hours and 30 minutes | Servings: 6

Ingredients:
- 4 cups low sodium veggie stock
- 28 ounces canned tomatoes, no-salt-added and crushed
- 1 teaspoon thyme, dried
- 1 teaspoon basil, dried
- ¼ teaspoon red pepper flakes
- A pinch of cayenne pepper
- 1 pound sweet potatoes, peeled and cubed
- 1 small yellow onion, chopped
- 1 teaspoon cilantro, dried
- Black pepper to the taste
- 1 pound scallops
- 1 pound shrimp, peeled and deveined

Directions:
1. Put tomatoes in your slow cooker; add garlic, sweet potatoes, stock, onion, cilantro, thyme, basil, pepper, cayenne and pepper flakes, stir, cover and cook on High for 3 hours.
2. Add scallops and shrimp, stir gently, cover, cook on High for 30 minutes more, divide into bowls and serve.

Nutrition: Calories 306, Fat 3.3g, Cholesterol 184mg, Sodium 767mg, Carbohydrate 35.9g, Fiber 5.1g, Sugars 6.5g, Protein 32.6g, Potassium 1323mg

Chicken and Potatoes

Preparation time: 10 minutes | Cooking time: 6 hours | Servings: 4

Ingredients:
- 1 pound chicken breast, skinless, boneless and cubed
- ½ pound sweet potatoes, peeled and cut into wedges
- 1 teaspoon coriander, ground
- 1 red onion, sliced
- 1 carrot, peeled and sliced
- 1 cup low-sodium chicken stock
- 1 teaspoon hot paprika
- ½ cup tomato juice
- 2 teaspoons olive oil
- A pinch of black pepper
- 2 garlic cloves, minced

Directions:
1. In your slow cooker, combine the chicken with the potatoes, coriander and the other ingredients, put the lid on and cook on Low for 6 hours.
2. Stir the whole mix once again, divide it between plates and serve.

Nutrition: Calories 246, Fat 5.3g, Cholesterol 73mg, Sodium 193mg, Carbohydrate 22.1g, Fiber 3.5g, Sugars 3.4g, Protein 26.2g, Potassium 1048mg

Slow Cooked Tuna

Preparation time: 10 minutes | Cooking time: 4 hours and 10 minutes | Servings: 2

Ingredients:
- 2 teaspoons black peppercorns, ground
- ½ pound tuna loin, cubed
- 1 cup olive oil
- 3 red chili peppers, chopped
- 1 garlic clove, minced
- 4 jalapeno peppers, chopped
- Black pepper to the taste

Directions:
1. Put the oil in your slow cooker; add chili peppers, jalapenos, peppercorns, pepper and garlic, whisk, cover and cook on Low for 4 hours.
2. Add tuna, toss, cook on High for 10 minutes more, divide between plates and serve.

Nutrition: Calories 1146, Fat 112.5g, Cholesterol 43mg, Sodium 1355mg, Carbohydrate 13g, Fiber 2.2g, Sugars 5.8g, Protein 29.7g, Potassium 131mg

Herbed Salmon

Preparation time: 10 minutes | Cooking time: 2 hours and 30 minutes | Servings: 4

Ingredients:
- 2 garlic cloves, minced
- 3 tablespoons lime juice
- 1 tablespoon olive oil
- 1 cup cilantro, chopped
- 4 salmon fillets,

boneless and skin on
- Black pepper to the taste

Directions:
1. Grease your slow cooker with the oil, place salmon fillets inside, add garlic, cilantro, lime juice and pepper, cover and cook on Low for 2 hours and 30 minutes.
2. Divide salmon between plates, drizzle the cilantro sauce from the slow cooker all over and serve.

Nutrition: Calories 305, Fat 16g, Cholesterol 78mg, Sodium 361mg, Carbohydrate 6.1g, Fiber 0.3g, Sugars 2.5g, Protein 35g, Potassium 727mg

Green Beans Soup

Preparation time: 10 minutes | Cooking time: 2 hours | Servings: 4

Ingredients:
- 2 pounds green beans, trimmed and halved
- 2 garlic cloves, minced
- 1 yellow onion, chopped
- 6 cups low-sodium chicken stock
- ½ cup tomato sauce, no-salt-added
- 1 tablespoon avocado oil
- 1 tablespoon basil, dried
- 1 tablespoon chives, chopped
- A pinch of black pepper

Directions:
1. In your slow cooker, combine the green beans with the garlic, onion and the other ingredients, put the lid on and cook on High for 2 hours.
2. Divide the soup into bowls and serve.

Nutrition: Calories 104, Fat 0.8g, Cholesterol 0mg, Sodium 218mg, Carbohydrate 21.2g, Fiber 9g, Sugars 5.7g, Protein 6.5g, Potassium 637mg

Coconut Clams

Preparation time: 10 minutes | Cooking time: 6 hours | Servings: 4

Ingredients:
- 21 ounces canned clams, no-salt-added, drained and chopped
- 2 tablespoons olive oil
- 4 eggs, whisked
- 1/3 cup green bell pepper, chopped
- ½ cup yellow onion, chopped
- Black pepper to the taste
- 1/3 cup coconut milk

Directions:
1. Put clams in your slow cooker, add milk, eggs, oil, onion, bell pepper and black pepper, toss, cover, cook on Low for 6 hours,

divide into bowls and serve.

Nutrition: Calories 282, Fat 18g, Cholesterol 164mg, Sodium 884mg, Carbohydrate 24.1g, Fiber 1.6g, Sugars 9.3g, Protein 7.4g, Potassium 284mg

Beef and Carrots

Preparation time: 10 minutes | Cooking time: 7 hours | Servings: 4

Ingredients:
- 2 pounds beef stew meat, cubed and browned
- 4 carrots, peeled and cubed
- 1 cup cherry tomatoes, halved
- 3 garlic cloves, minced
- 1 yellow onion, chopped
- 1 and ½ cups beef stock, low-sodium
- 1 teaspoon rosemary, dried
- 2 tablespoons cilantro, chopped

Directions:
1. In your slow cooker, combine the beef with the carrots, tomatoes and the other ingredients, put the lid on and cook on Low for 7 hours.
2. Divide the mix bowls and serve.

Nutrition: Calories 470, Fat 14.3g, Cholesterol 203 mg, Sodium 195mg, Carbohydrate 11.3g, Fiber 2.8g, Sugars 5.4g, Protein 70.2g, Potassium 1270mg

Creamy Seafood and Veggies Soup

Preparation time: 10 minutes | Cooking time: 3 hours | Servings: 12

Ingredients:
- 4 tilapia fillets, skinless, boneless and cubed
- 10 ounces coconut cream
- 2 cups low-sodium veggie stock
- 2 cups no-salt-added tomato sauce
- 12 ounces canned crab meat, no-salt-added and drained
- 2 celery stalks, chopped
- 3 kale stalks, chopped
- 1 bay leaf
- 1 and ½ cups water
- 1 and ½ pounds jumbo shrimp, peeled and deveined
- 1 yellow onion, chopped
- ½ teaspoon cloves, ground
- 1 teaspoon rosemary, dried
- 1 cup carrots, chopped
- 2 garlic cloves, minced
- 1 teaspoon thyme, dried

Directions:
1. In your slow cooker, mix coconut cream with stock, tomato sauce and water and stir.
2. Add shrimp, fish, onion, carrots, celery, kale, garlic, bay leaf, cloves, thyme and rosemary,

cover, cook on Low for 3 hours, stir, ladle into bowls and serve.

Nutrition: Calories 184, Fat 6.6g, Cholesterol 150mg, Sodium 1109mg, Carbohydrate 8.8g, Fiber 2.1g, Sugars 4.6g, Protein 22.6g, Potassium 357mg

Beef Chili Mix

Preparation time: 10 minutes | Cooking time: 4 hours | Servings: 4

Ingredients:
- 1 cup low-sodium beef stock
- 2 pounds beef meat, ground and browned
- 1 red onion, sliced
- 1 red bell pepper, chopped
- 1 cup corn
- 1 cup cherry tomatoes, halved
- 1 teaspoon rosemary, dried
- 2 tablespoons tomato juice
- 1 tablespoon avocado oil
- 3 garlic cloves, minced
- 1 tablespoon chili powder
- A pinch of black pepper

Directions:
1. In your slow cooker, combine the beef with the stock, onion and the other ingredients, put the lid on and cook on High for 4 hours.
2. Divide the chili into bowls and serve hot.

Nutrition: Calories 518, Fat 8.1g, Cholesterol 202 mg, Sodium 278mg, Carbohydrate 16.3g, Fiber 3.6g, Sugars 5.5g, Protein 69.4g, Potassium 1278mg

Seafood Gumbo

Preparation time: 10 minutes | Cooking time: 6 hours | Servings: 4

Ingredients:
- 10 ounces canned tomato paste, no-salt-added
- 1 pound shrimp, peeled and deveined
- 1 yellow onion, chopped
- 2 pounds mussels, cleaned and debearded
- 28 ounces canned clams, no-salt-added and drained

Directions:
1. In your slow cooker, mix shrimp with mussels, clams, onion and tomato paste, stir, cover, cook on Low for 6 hours, divide into bowls and serve.

Nutrition: Calories 494, Fat 7.8g, Cholesterol 302mg, Sodium 1714mg, Carbohydrate 47.8g, Fiber 4.3g, Sugars 16.4g, Protein 18.4g, Potassium 1853mg

Lemon and Spinach Trout

Preparation time: 10 minutes | Cooking time: 2 hours | Servings: 4

Ingredients:
- 12 ounces spinach
- 2 lemons, sliced
- ¼ cup low sodium chicken stock
- 2 tablespoons dill, chopped
- Black pepper to the taste
- 4 medium trout

Directions:
1. Put the stock in your slow cooker and add the fish inside
2. Season with black pepper to the taste, top with lemon slices, dill and spinach, cover and cook on High for 2 hours.
3. Divide fish, lemon and spinach between plates and serve.

Nutrition: Calories 227, Fat 9.2g, Cholesterol 62mg, Sodium 412mg, Carbohydrate 11g, Fiber 3g, Sugars 3.3g, Protein 26.1g, Potassium 959mg

Lentils and Shrimp Soup

Preparation time: 10 minutes | Cooking time: 2 hours and 30 minutes | Servings: 4

Ingredients:
- 2 teaspoons avocado oil
- 1 pound shrimp, peeled and deveined
- 1 and ½ cups canned lentils, no-salt added, drained and rinsed
- 1 red onion, chopped
- 1 celery stalk, chopped
- 4 garlic cloves, minced
- 1 teaspoon thyme, dried
- 6 cups low-sodium chicken stock
- 1 teaspoon sweet paprika
- 1 tablespoon chives, chopped

Directions:
1. In your slow cooker, mix the shrimp with the lentils, onion and the other ingredients, put the lid on and cook on High for 2 hours and 30 minutes.
2. Ladle the soup into bowls and serve.

Nutrition: Calories 213, Fat 2.4g, Cholesterol 239mg, Sodium 455mg, Carbohydrate 15.9g, Fiber 5.5g, Sugars 2.3g, Protein 33.5g, Potassium 277mg

Mexican Chicken

Preparation time: 10 minutes | Cooking time: 7 hours | Servings: 4

Ingredients:
- 4 chicken breasts, skinless and boneless
- 1 teaspoon chili powder
- ½ cup water
- 16 ounces chunky salsa
- 1 and ½ tablespoons parsley, chopped
- 1 teaspoon garlic powder
- ½ teaspoon sweet

- paprika
- ½ tablespoon cilantro, chopped
- 1 teaspoon onion powder
- ½ tablespoons oregano, dried
- ½ teaspoon cumin, ground
- Black pepper to the taste

Directions:
1. Put the water in your slow cooker, add chicken breasts, salsa, parsley, garlic powder, cilantro, onion powder, oregano, paprika, chili powder, cumin and black pepper to the taste, toss, cover and cook on Low for 7 hours.
2. Divide the whole mix between plates and serve.

Nutrition: Calories 435, Fat 16.1g, Cholesterol 169mg, Sodium 1133mg, Carbohydrate 13.4g, Fiber 2.7g, Sugars 6.2g, Protein 57.4g, Potassium 853mg

Oregano Turkey Mix

Preparation time: 10 minutes | Cooking time: 4 hours | Servings: 4

Ingredients:
- 2 pounds turkey breast, skinless, boneless and sliced
- 2 teaspoons sweet paprika
- 1 tablespoon oregano, chopped
- 2 tablespoons avocado oil
- 1 yellow onion, chopped
- 1 red bell pepper, chopped
- ¼ teaspoon red pepper flakes, crushed
- 1 cup canned tomatoes, no-salt-added, crushed
- 1 tablespoon chives, chopped

Directions:
1. In your slow cooker, combine the turkey with the paprika, oregano and the other ingredients, put the lid on and cook on High for 4 hours.
2. Divide the whole mix between plates and serve.

Nutrition: Calories 281, Fat 5.1g, Cholesterol 98mg, Sodium 2307mg, Carbohydrate 17.9g, Fiber 3.9g, Sugars 12g, Protein 40.1g, Potassium 958mg

Chicken Breast Stew

Preparation time: 10 minutes | Cooking time: 8 hours | Servings: 4

Ingredients:
- 1 yellow onion, chopped
- 2 pounds chicken breasts, skinless and boneless
- 4 ounces canned jalapenos, drained and chopped
- 3 garlic cloves, minced
- 1 tablespoon chili powder
- 4 ounces canned green chilies, drained and chopped
- 7 ounces tomato sauce
- 14 ounces canned tomatoes, chopped
- 2 teaspoons oregano, dried
- 2 tablespoons coconut oil, melted
- 1 tablespoon cumin, ground
- Black pepper to the taste
- 1 green bell pepper, chopped
- 1 avocado, pitted, peeled and sliced
- A bunch of cilantro, chopped

Directions:
1. Grease the slow cooker with the melted oil, add onion, chicken, jalapenos, bell pepper, green chilies, tomato sauce, tomatoes, garlic, chili powder, cumin, oregano and black pepper, stir, cover and cook on Low for 8 hours.
2. Add cilantro, shred chicken breasts using 2 forks, stir the stew, divide into bowls and top with avocado slices.

Nutrition: Calories 768, Fat 36.7g, Cholesterol 202mg, Sodium 571mg, Carbohydrate 41.1g, Fiber 16.6g, Sugars 21g, Protein 72.9g, Potassium 1992mg

Turkey Breast and Sweet Potato Mix

Preparation time: 10 minutes | Cooking time: 8 hours | Servings: 4

Ingredients:
- 3 sweet potatoes, cut into wedges
- 3 pounds turkey breast, bone in
- 1/3 cup water
- 1 cup dried cherries, pitted
- 2 white onions, cut into wedges
- 1 teaspoon thyme, dried
- 1 teaspoon sage, dried
- 1 teaspoon onion powder
- 1 teaspoon garlic powder
- 1 teaspoon parsley flakes
- 1 teaspoon paprika, dried
- Black pepper to the taste

Directions:
1. Put the turkey breast in your slow cooker, add sweet potatoes, cherries, onions, water, parsley, garlic and onion powder, thyme, sage, paprika and pepper, toss, cover and cook on Low for 8 hours.
2. Discard bone from turkey breast, slice meat and divide between plates.
3. Serve with the veggies and the cherries on the side.

Nutrition: Calories 439, Fat 6.2g, Cholesterol 146mg, Sodium 3534mg, Carbohydrate 33.6g, Fiber 4.5g, Sugars 16.5g, Protein 59.6g, Potassium 1268mg

Creamy Pork Chops

Preparation time: 10 minutes | Cooking time: 6 hours | Servings: 4

Ingredients:
- 2 pound pork chops, browned
- 4 spring onions, chopped
- 3 garlic cloves, minced
- 1 cup coconut cream
- 1 tablespoon balsamic vinegar
- 1 tablespoon olive oil
- 1 teaspoon chili powder
- A pinch of black pepper
- 1 teaspoon sweet paprika

Directions:
1. In the slow cooker, combine the pork chops with the spring onions, garlic and the other ingredients, put the lid on and cook on Low for 6 hours.
2. Toss, divide between plates and serve.

Nutrition: Calories 906, Fat 74.4g, Cholesterol 195mg, Sodium 177mg, Carbohydrate 5.9g, Fiber 2.2g, Sugars 2.5g, Protein 52.9g, Potassium 1016mg

Italian Chicken

Preparation time: 10 minutes | Cooking time: 5 hours | Servings: 4

Ingredients:
- 4 chicken breasts, skinless and boneless
- 29 ounces canned tomatoes, chopped
- 15 ounces tomato sauce, no-salt-added
- 6 Italian sausages, sliced
- 1 white onion, chopped
- 5 garlic cloves, minced
- 1 teaspoon Italian seasoning
- A drizzle of olive oil
- 1 cup water
- 1 teaspoon garlic powder
- ½ cup balsamic vinegar

Directions:
1. Put chicken and sausage slices in your slow cooker, add garlic, onion, Italian seasoning, the oil, tomatoes, tomato sauce, garlic powder, water and the vinegar, cover and cook on High for 5 hours.
2. Stir chicken and sausage mix, divide between plates and serve.

Nutrition: Calories 864, Fat 55.5g, Cholesterol 238mg, Sodium 1699mg, Carbohydrate 21g, Fiber 45.5g, Sugars 12.8g, Protein 67.2g, Potassium 1635mg

Chicken Breast and Cinnamon Veggie Mix

Preparation time: 10 minutes | Cooking time: 6 hours | Servings: 4

Ingredients:
- 4 garlic cloves, minced
- 2 red bell peppers, chopped
- 2 pounds chicken breasts, skinless and boneless
- 1 cup low sodium chicken stock
- 1 yellow onion, chopped
- 2 teaspoons cinnamon powder
- ¼ teaspoon nutmeg, ground
- 2 teaspoons paprika

Directions:
1. In a bowl, mix bell peppers with chicken breasts, garlic, onion, paprika, cinnamon and nutmeg, toss to coat, transfer everything to your slow cooker, add stock, cover, cook on Low for 6 hours, divide everything between plates and serve.

Nutrition: Calories 473, Fat 17.2g, Cholesterol 202mg, Sodium 216mg, Carbohydrate 9g, Fiber 1.9g, Sugars 4.4g, Protein 67.4g, Potassium 740mg

Paprika Pork and Broccoli

Preparation time: 10 minutes | Cooking time: 6 hours | Servings: 4

Ingredients:
- ½ cup beef stock, low-sodium
- 2 pounds pork stew meat, cubed
- ½ pound broccoli florets
- 1 cup tomato juice
- 1 tablespoon olive oil
- 1 teaspoon smoked paprika
- 1 teaspoon garam masala
- 1 teaspoon coriander, ground

Directions:
1. In the slow cooker, combine the meat with the stock, broccoli and the other ingredients, put the lid on and cook on Low for 6 hours.
2. Divide the mix between plates and serve

Nutrition: Calories 543, Fat 25.7g, Cholesterol 195mg, Sodium 335mg, Carbohydrate 6.6g, Fiber 1.9g, Sugars 3.2g, Protein 68.8g, Potassium 1182mg

Mexican Beef Mix

Preparation time: 10 minutes | Cooking time: 8 hours and 3 minutes | Servings: 6

Ingredients:
- 5 pounds beef roast
- 1 yellow onion, chopped
- 2 tablespoons sweet paprika
- 15 ounces canned tomatoes, no-salt-added, roasted and chopped

- Juice of 1 lemon
- 1 teaspoon cumin, ground
- 1 teaspoon olive oil
- A pinch of nutmeg,
- ground
- ¼ cup apple cider vinegar
- Black pepper to the taste

Directions:
1. Heat up a pan with the oil over medium-high heat, add onions, stir, brown them for 2-3 minutes, transfer them to your slow cooker, add paprika, tomato, cumin, nutmeg, lemon juice, vinegar, black pepper and beef, toss to coat, cover and cook on Low for 8 hours.
2. Slice roast, divide between plates and serve with tomatoes and onions mix on the side.

Nutrition: Calories 744, Fat 25.1g, Cholesterol 338mg, Sodium 285mg, Carbohydrate 6.6g, Fiber 2.2g, Sugars 4.4g, Protein 3.3g, Potassium 1795mg

Maple Beef Tenderloin

Preparation time: 10 minutes | Cooking time: 8 hours | Servings: 4

Ingredients:
- 2 pounds beef tenderloin, trimmed
- 2 tablespoons maple syrup
- 4 apples, cored and sliced
- A pinch of nutmeg, ground

Directions:
1. Place half of the apples in your slow cooker, sprinkle the nutmeg over them, add beef tenderloin, top with the rest of the apples, drizzle the maple syrup, cover and cook on Low for 8 hours.
2. Slice beef tenderloin, divide between plates and serve with apple slices and cooking juices on top.

Nutrition: Calories 610, Fat 21.2g, Cholesterol 209mg, Sodium 137mg, Carbohydrate 37.5g, Fiber 5.4g, Sugars 29.2g, Protein 66.3g, Potassium 1069mg

Mushroom Cream

Preparation time: 10 minutes | Cooking time: 3 hours | Servings: 4

Ingredients:
- 1 pound mushrooms, sliced
- 4 cups low-sodium chicken stock
- 1 cup coconut cream
- 1 teaspoon turmeric powder
- A pinch of black pepper
- ¼ teaspoon garlic powder
- ½ teaspoon onion powder
- 2 teaspoons olive oil
- 1 yellow onion, chopped
- 1 tablespoon chives, chopped

Directions:
1. In the slow cooker, combine the mushrooms with the stock, turmeric and the other ingredients except the cream, put the lid on and cook on High for 3 hours.
2. Add the cream, blend using an immersion blender, ladle into bowls, and serve.

Nutrition: Calories 212, Fat 17g, Cholesterol 0mg, Sodium 87mg, Carbohydrate 11.4g, Fiber 3.2g, Sugars 5.3g, Protein 7.3g, Potassium 580mg

Beef and Cabbage Stew

Preparation time: 10 minutes | Cooking time: 8 hours and 10 minutes | Servings: 6

Ingredients:
- 1 tablespoon olive oil
- 2 pounds beef loin, cubed
- 28 ounces canned tomatoes, no-salt-added, drained and chopped
- 3 garlic cloves, minced
- 2 onions, chopped
- 6 baby carrots, halved
- 1 cabbage head, shredded
- 3 cups veggie stock
- 3 big sweet potatoes, cubed
- Black pepper to the taste

Directions:
1. Heat up a pan with the oil over medium-high heat, add meat, brown for a few minutes on each side, transfer to your slow cooker, add black pepper, carrots, garlic, onion, potatoes, cabbage, stock and tomatoes, stir well, cover, cook on Low for 8 hours, divide the stew into bowls and serve right away.

Nutrition: Calories 610, Fat 21.2g, Cholesterol 209mg, Sodium 137mg, Carbohydrate 37.5g, Fiber 5.4g, Sugars 29.2g, Protein 66.3g, Potassium 1069mg

Greek Beef

Preparation time: 1 day | Cooking time: 8 hours | Servings: 6

Ingredients:
- 3 pounds beef shoulder, boneless
- 2 teaspoons oregano, dried
- 6 garlic cloves, minced
- 2 teaspoons mustard
- 2 teaspoons mint
- ¼ cup olive oil
- ¼ cup lemon juice
- Black pepper to the taste

Directions:
1. In a bowl, mix oil with lemon juice, oregano, mint, mustard, garlic and pepper, whisk, rub the meat with the marinade, cover and keep in the fridge for 1 day.

2. Transfer to your slow cooker along with the marinade, cover, cook on Low for 8 hours, slice the roast and serve.

Nutrition: Calories 610, Fat 21.2g, Cholesterol 209mg, Sodium 137mg, Carbohydrate 37.5g, Fiber 5.4g, Sugars 29.2g, Protein 66.3g, Potassium 1069mg

Garlic Chicken Mix

Preparation time: 10 minutes | Cooking time: 6 hours | Servings: 4

Ingredients:
- 2 pounds chicken thighs, skinless, boneless and cubed
- 2 tablespoons avocado oil
- 5 garlic cloves, minced
- 1 cup cherry tomatoes, halved
- 1 cup low sodium chicken stock
- 2 green chilies, chopped
- Black pepper to the taste
- 1 teaspoon cinnamon, ground
- 1 teaspoon turmeric powder
- Juice of 1 lime

Directions:
1. In your slow cooker, combine the chicken with the oil, garlic and the other ingredients, put the lid on and cook on Low for 6 hours.
2. Divide the mix into bowls and serve.

Nutrition: Calories 465, Fat 17.9g, Cholesterol 202mg, Sodium 216mg, Carbohydrate 5.6g, Fiber 1.5g, Sugars 1.6g, Protein 67g, Potassium 729mg

Roast and Veggies

Preparation time: 10 minutes | Cooking time: 4 hours | Servings: 6

Ingredients:
- 1 pound sweet potatoes, chopped
- 15 ounces canned tomatoes, no-salt-added and chopped
- 3 and ½ pounds beef roast, trimmed
- 8 medium carrots, chopped
- Juice of 1 lemon
- 1 yellow onion, chopped
- 4 garlic cloves, minced
- Zest of 1 lemon, grated
- Black pepper to the taste
- ½ cup kalamata olives, pitted

Directions:
1. Put potatoes in your slow cooker, carrots, tomatoes, onions, lemon juice and zest, beef, black pepper and garlic, stir, cover and cook on High for 4 hours.
2. Transfer meat to a cutting board, slice it and divide between plates.
3. Transfer the veggies to a bowl, mash, mix them with olives, and add next to the meat.

Nutrition: Calories 659, Fat 18.3g, Cholesterol 236mg, Sodium 378mg, Carbohydrate 36.5g, Fiber 7.1g, Sugars 7.7g, Protein 83.3g, Potassium 2169mg

Beef Roast Soup

Preparation time: 10 minutes | Cooking time: 7 hours | Servings: 4

Ingredients:
- 4 thyme springs
- 2 pounds beef roast
- 6 red onions, sliced
- 1 bay leaf
- 2 quarts low sodium veggie stock
- ½ cup sherry vinegar
- A pinch of black pepper
- 2 tablespoons olive oil

Directions:
1. In your slow cooker, mix the roast with stock, bay leaf and thyme, cover, cook on High for 6 hours, transfer roast to a cutting board, shred and transfer to a bowl.
2. Heat up a large pot with the oil over medium-high heat, add onions, stir, cook them for 5 minutes and transfer to your slow cooker,
3. Add vinegar, some pepper and return the meat, stir, cover, cook for 45 minutes more, ladle into bowls and serve.

Nutrition: Calories 579, Fat 21.3g, Cholesterol 203mg, Sodium 436mg, Carbohydrate 20g, Fiber 3.7g, Sugars 9g, Protein 70.7g, Potassium 1160mg

Cod Soup

Preparation time: 10 minutes | Cooking time: 2 hours | Servings: 4

Ingredients:
- 1 red onion, chopped
- 6 cups low-sodium chicken stock
- 1 pound cod fillets, boneless and cubed
- 1 zucchini, cubed
- ½ cup cherry tomatoes, halved
- 1 carrot, peeled and sliced
- 1 tablespoon olive oil
- Black pepper to the taste
- 2 tablespoons cilantro, chopped

Directions:
1. In the slow cooker, combine the fish with the stock, zucchini and the other ingredients, put the lid on and cook on Low for 2 hours.
2. Toss the soup gently, ladle into bowls and serve hot.

Nutrition: Calories 205, Fat 6.2g, Cholesterol 56mg, Sodium 474mg, Carbohydrate 12.4g, Fiber 1.9g, Sugars 5.6g, Protein 24.7g, Potassium 273mg

Coconut Salmon Soup

Preparation time: 10 minutes | Cooking time: 4 hours | Servings: 6

Ingredients:
- 2 tablespoons olive oil
- 6 cups low sodium chicken stock
- 4 leeks, sliced
- 3 garlic cloves, minced
- 2 teaspoons thyme, dried
- 1 and ¼ cup coconut milk
- 1 pounds salmon, skinless, boneless and cubed
- A pinch of black pepper

Directions:
1. Heat up a pan with the oil over medium-high heat, add garlic and leeks, stir, brown for a few minutes, transfer them to your slow cooker, add stock, thyme and pepper, cover and cook on Low for 3 hours.
2. Add coconut milk and salmon, cover, cook on Low for 1 hour, ladle into bowls and serve.

Nutrition: Calories 309, Fat 21.5g, Cholesterol 33mg, Sodium 123mg, Carbohydrate 12.9g, Fiber 2.3g, Sugars 4g, Protein 18.8g, Potassium 538mg

Ground Beef and Veggies Soup

Preparation time: 10 minutes | Cooking time: 6 hours and 10 minutes | Servings: 4

Ingredients:
- 1 pound beef, ground
- 1 carrot, chopped
- 3 cups water
- 2 zucchinis, chopped
- 1 yellow onion, chopped
- 29 ounces canned tomatoes, no-salt-added and chopped
- 1 celery stalk, chopped
- ½ cup low sodium veggie stock
- A pinch of black pepper
- 1 tablespoon garlic, minced
- ½ teaspoon oregano, dried
- ½ teaspoon basil, dried

Directions:
1. Heat up a pan over medium-high heat, add meat, brown for a few minutes, transfer to your slow cooker, add water, zucchinis, carrot, onion, celery, stock, pepper, tomatoes, garlic, oregano and basil, stir, cover, cook on Low for 6 hours, ladle into bowls and serve.

Nutrition: Calories 287, Fat 7.7g, Cholesterol 101mg, Sodium 133mg, Carbohydrate 16.6g, Fiber 4.7g, Sugars 9.3g, Protein 38g, Potassium 1315mg

Shrimp and Asparagus

Preparation time: 10 minutes | Cooking time: 2 hours | Servings: 4

Ingredients:
- 1 pound shrimp, peeled and deveined
- 1 red onion, chopped
- 8 asparagus spears, cut into medium pieces
- Black pepper to the taste
- 2 teaspoons olive oil
- ½ teaspoon coriander, ground
- ½ teaspoon rosemary, dried
- 1 teaspoon red pepper flakes, crushed
- 2 garlic cloves, minced
- 1 cup low-sodium veggie stock
- 1 tablespoon chives, chopped

Directions:
1. In the slow cooker, combine the shrimp with the onion, asparagus and the other ingredients, put the lid on and cook on High for 2 hours.
2. Divide everything between plates and serve.

Nutrition: Calories 184, Fat 4.5g, Cholesterol 239mg, Sodium 377mg, Carbohydrate 8.1g, Fiber 1.8g, Sugars 2.4g, Protein 27.4g, Potassium 349mg

Greek Cod Mix

Preparation time: 10 minutes | Cooking time: 2 hours | Servings: 4

Ingredients:
- 4 cod fillets, boneless and skinless
- 1 cup black olives, pitted and chopped
- 1 tablespoon olive oil
- 1 pound cherry tomatoes, halved
- 1 garlic clove, minced
- ½ cup low sodium veggie stock
- A pinch of black pepper
- A pinch of thyme, dried

Directions:
1. In your slow cooker, mix cod with black olives, oil, garlic, stock, pepper, cherry tomatoes and thyme, cover, cook on High for 2 hours, divide everything between plates and serve.

Nutrition: Calories 182, Fat 8.3g, Cholesterol 40mg, Sodium 396mg, Carbohydrate 7.1g, Fiber 2.5g, Sugars 3.1g, Protein 21.3g, Potassium 275mg

Creamy Fish Curry

Preparation time: 10 minutes | Cooking time: 2 hours | Servings: 6

Ingredients:
- 6 cod fillets, skinless, boneless and cubed
- 6 curry leaves
- 1 tomato, chopped
- 14 ounces coconut milk, unsweetened
- 2 yellow onions, sliced
- 2 green bell peppers, chopped

- 2 garlic cloves, minced
- 2 teaspoons cumin, ground
- 2 tablespoons lemon juice
- ½ teaspoon turmeric powder
- A pinch of black pepper
- 1 tablespoons coriander, ground
- 1 tablespoon ginger, grated

Directions:

1. In your slow cooker, mix fish with tomato, coconut milk, onions, green bell peppers, garlic, curry leaves, turmeric, pepper, cumin, lemon juice, coriander and ginger, toss, cover, cook on High for 2 hours, divide into bowls and serve.

Nutrition: Calories 287, Fat 17.5g, Cholesterol 55mg, Sodium 87mg, Carbohydrate 13.2g, Fiber 3.8g, Sugars 6.3g, Protein 23g, Potassium 398mg

Hot Mackerel

Preparation time: 10 minutes | Cooking time: 2 hours and 30 minutes | Servings: 4

Ingredients:

- 18 ounces mackerel, skinless, boneless and cut into pieces
- 2 lemongrass sticks, halved
- 3 garlic cloves, minced
- 8 shallots, chopped
- 3 and ½ ounces water
- 5 tablespoons olive oil
- 1 ginger slice, grated
- 1 teaspoon turmeric powder
- 1 tablespoon chili paste
- 1 and 1/3 tablespoons tamarind paste

Directions:

1. In your blender, mix garlic with shallots, chili paste and turmeric, blend well and add to slow cooker.
2. Add fish, oil, ginger, lemongrass, tamarind and water, stir, cover, cook on Low for 2 hours and 30 minutes, divide between plates and serve.

Nutrition: Calories 526, Fat 41g, Cholesterol 97mg, Sodium 156mg, Carbohydrate 8.5g, Fiber 0.4g, Sugars 2.5g, Protein 31.5g, Potassium 641mg

Lemon and Basil Sea Bass

Preparation time: 10 minutes | Cooking time: 2 hours | Servings: 4

Ingredients:

- 2 tablespoons avocado oil
- 2 pounds sea bass fillets, boneless
- Juice of 1 lemon
- 2 tablespoons lemon zest, grated
- Black pepper to the taste
- 1 tablespoon basil, chopped
- ½ cup low-sodium chicken stock

Directions:

1. In the slow cooker, combine the sea bass with the oil, lemon juice and the other ingredients, put the lid on and cook on High for 2 hours.
2. Toss the mix, divide between plates and serve.

Nutrition: Calories 296, Fat 6.8g, Cholesterol 120mg, Sodium 217mg, Carbohydrate 1.3g, Fiber 0.6g, Sugars 0.4g, Protein 54g, Potassium 792mg

Mussels Mix

Preparation time: 10 minutes | Cooking time: 2 hours | Servings: 4

Ingredients:

- 2 pounds mussels, scrubbed
- 2 teaspoons garlic, minced
- 2 tablespoons olive oil
- 1 yellow onion, chopped
- 14 ounces canned tomatoes, no-salt-added and chopped
- 1 teaspoon parsley, dried
- ½ teaspoon red pepper flakes, crushed
- ½ cup low sodium chicken stock

Directions:

1. In your slow cooker, mix mussels with oil, onion parsley, pepper flakes, garlic, tomatoes and stock, stir, cover, cook on High for 2 hours, divide into bowls and serve.

Nutrition: Calories 289, Fat 12.4g, Cholesterol 64mg, Sodium 664mg, Carbohydrate 15.5g, Fiber 1.9g, Sugars 3.8g, Protein 28.5g, Potassium 1013mg

Turkey Wings and Veggies

Preparation time: 10 minutes | Cooking time: 8 hours | Servings: 4

Ingredients:

- 3 garlic cloves, minced
- 4 turkey wings
- 1 yellow onion, chopped
- 1 carrot, chopped
- 1 celery stalk, chopped
- 2 tablespoons olive oil
- A pinch of sage, dried
- A pinch of thyme, dried
- 1 cup low sodium chicken stock
- Black pepper to the taste
- 1 teaspoon rosemary, dried

Directions:

1. In your slow cooker, mix turkey wings with the onion, carrot, garlic, celery, stock, black pepper, oil, rosemary, sage and thyme, toss, cover, cook on Low for 8 hours, divide between plates and serve.

Nutrition: Calories 273, Fat 17.3g, Cholesterol 0mg, Sodium 75mg, Carbohydrate 6.1g, Fiber 1.3g, Sugars 2.3g, Protein 24.2g, Potassium 112mg

Pork Chops and Cabbage

Preparation time: 10 minutes | Cooking time: 4 hours | Servings: 4

Ingredients:
- 2 pounds pork chops
- 1 green cabbage head, shredded
- 1 cup tomato sauce
- 1 teaspoon mustard seeds, crushed
- 1 bay leaf
- 3 garlic cloves, chopped
- 1 teaspoon sweet paprika
- Black pepper to the taste

Directions:
1. In the slow cooker, combine the pork chops with the cabbage, tomato sauce and other ingredients, put the lid on and cook on High for 4 hours.
2. Divide between plates and serve.

Nutrition: Calories 795, Fat 57g, Cholesterol 195mg, Sodium 513mg, Carbohydrate 15.2g, Fiber 5.8g, Sugars 8.4g, Protein 54.5g, Potassium 1315mg

Citrus Turkey Mix

Preparation time: 10 minutes | Cooking time: 8 hours | Servings: 4

Ingredients:
- 4 turkey wings
- 1 and ½ cups cranberries, dried
- 1 cup walnuts, chopped
- 1 cup orange juice
- 2 tablespoons olive oil
- Black pepper to the taste
- 1 yellow onion, chopped
- 1 bunch thyme, chopped

Directions:
1. Grease the slow cooker with the oil, add turkey wings, cranberries, pepper, onion, walnuts, orange juice and thyme, cover, cook on Low for 8 hours, divide everything between plates and serve.

Nutrition: Calories 504, Fat 35.9g, Cholesterol 0mg, Sodium 58mg, Carbohydrate 16.9g, Fiber 4.5g, Sugars 8.7g, Protein 31.3g, Potassium 400mg

Dash Diet Slow Cooker Side Dish Recipes

Zucchini and Sprouts Salad

Preparation time: 10 minutes | Cooking time: 3 hours | Servings: 4

Ingredients:
- 1 pound zucchinis, roughly cubed
- ½ pound Brussels sprouts, trimmed and halved
- ¼ cup veggie stock, low-sodium
- 1 teaspoon cumin, ground
- 1 teaspoon chili powder
- 2 teaspoons avocado oil

Directions:
1. In slow cooker, combine the sprouts with the zucchinis and the other ingredients, put the lid on and cook on Low for 3 hours.
2. Divide between plates and serve as a side dish.

Nutrition: Calories 51, Fat 0.9g, Cholesterol 0mg, Sodium 42mg, Carbohydrate 9.8g, Fiber 3.8g, Sugars 3.3g, Protein 3.5g, Potassium 547mg

Broccoli Mix

Preparation time: 10 minutes | Cooking time: 3 hours | Servings: 10

Ingredients:
- 6 cups broccoli florets
- 1 and ½ cups low-fat cheddar cheese, shredded
- ½ teaspoon cider vinegar
- ¼ cup yellow onion, chopped
- 10 ounces tomato sauce, sodium-free
- 2 tablespoons olive oil
- A pinch of black pepper

Directions:
1. Grease your slow cooker with the oil, add broccoli, tomato sauce, cider vinegar, onion and black pepper, cover and cook on High for 2 hours and 30 minutes.
2. Sprinkle the cheese all over, cover, cook on High for 30 minutes more, divide between plates and serve as a side dish.

Nutrition: Calories 119, Fat 8.7g, Cholesterol 18mg, Sodium 272mg, Carbohydrate 5.7g, Fiber 1.9g, Sugars 2.3g, Protein 6.2g, Potassium 288mg

Tasty Bean Side Dish

Preparation time: 10 minutes | Cooking time: 5 hours | Servings: 10

Ingredients:
- 1 green bell pepper, chopped
- 1 sweet red pepper, chopped
- 1 and ½ cups tomato sauce, salt-free
- 1 yellow onion, chopped
- ½ cup water
- 16 ounces canned kidney beans, no-salt-added, drained

and rinsed
- 16 ounces canned black-eyed peas, no-salt-added, drained and rinsed
- 15 ounces corn
- 15 ounces canned lima beans, no-salt-added, drained and rinsed
- 15 ounces canned black beans, no-salt-added, drained and rinsed
- 2 celery ribs, chopped
- 2 bay leaves
- 1 teaspoon ground mustard
- 1 tablespoon cider vinegar

Directions:
1. In your slow cooker, mix the tomato sauce with the onion, celery, red pepper, green bell pepper, water, bay leaves, mustard, vinegar, kidney beans, black-eyed peas, corn, lima beans and black beans, cover and cook on Low for 5 hours.
2. Discard bay leaves, divide the whole mix between plates and serve.

Nutrition: Calories 602, Fat 4.8g, Cholesterol 0mg, Sodium 255mg, Carbohydrate 117.7g, Fiber 24.6g, Sugars 13.4g, Protein 33g, Potassium 2355mg

Green Beans

Preparation time: 10 minutes | Cooking time: 2 hours | Servings: 12

Ingredients:
- 3 tablespoons olive oil
- 16 ounces green beans
- ½ teaspoon garlic powder
- ½ cup coconut sugar
- 1 teaspoon low-sodium soy sauce

Directions:
1. In your slow cooker, mix the green beans with the oil, sugar, soy sauce and garlic powder, cover and cook on Low for 2 hours.
2. Toss the beans, divide them between plates and serve as a side dish.

Nutrition: Calories 46, Fat 3.6g, Cholesterol 0mg, Sodium 29mg, Carbohydrate 3.6g, Fiber 1.3g, Sugars 0.6g, Protein 0.8g, Potassium 80mg

Creamy Corn

Preparation time: 10 minutes | Cooking time: 4 hours | Servings: 12

Ingredients:
- 20 ounces fat-free cream cheese
- 10 cups corn
- ½ cup low-fat butter
- ½ cup fat-free milk
- A pinch of black pepper
- 2 tablespoons green onions, chopped

Directions:

1. In your slow cooker, mix the corn with cream cheese, milk, butter, black pepper and onions, toss, cover and cook on Low for 4 hours.
2. Toss one more time, divide between plates and serve as a side dish.

Nutrition: Calories 279, Fat 18g, Cholesterol 52mg, Sodium 165mg, Carbohydrate 26g, Fiber 3.5g, Sugars 4.8g, Protein 8.1g, Potassium 422mg

Classic Peas and Carrots

Preparation time: 10 minutes | Cooking time: 5 hours | Servings: 12

Ingredients:
- 1 pound carrots, sliced
- 1 yellow onion, chopped
- 16 ounces peas
- 2 tablespoons stevia
- 2 tablespoons olive oil
- 4 garlic cloves, minced
- ¼ cup water
- 1 teaspoon marjoram, dried
- A pinch of white pepper

Directions:
1. In your slow cooker, mix the carrots with water, onion, oil, stevia, garlic, marjoram, white pepper and peas, toss, cover and cook on High for 5 hours.
2. Divide between plates and serve as a side dish.

Nutrition: Calories 71, Fat 2.5g, Cholesterol 0mg, Sodium 29mg, Carbohydrate 12.1g, Fiber 3.1g, Sugars 4.4g, Protein 2.5g, Potassium 231mg

Mushroom Pilaf

Preparation time: 10 minutes | Cooking time: 3 hours | Servings: 6

Ingredients:
- 1 cup wild rice
- 6 green onions, chopped
- ½ pound baby Bella mushrooms
- 2 cups water
- 2 tablespoons olive oil
- 2 garlic cloves, minced

Directions:
1. In your slow cooker, mix the rice with garlic, onions, oil, mushrooms and water, toss, cover and cook on Low for 3 hours.
2. Stir the pilaf one more time, divide between plates and serve.

Nutrition: Calories 151, Fat 5.1g, Cholesterol 0mg, Sodium 9mg, Carbohydrate 23.3g, Fiber 2.6g, Sugars 1.7g, Protein 5.2g, Potassium 343mg

Lime Fennel

Preparation time: 10 minutes | Cooking time: 2 hours and 30 minutes | Servings: 4

Ingredients:
- 2 fennel bulbs, sliced
- Juice and zest of 1 lime
- 2 teaspoons avocado oil
- ½ teaspoon turmeric powder
- 1 tablespoon parsley, chopped
- ¼ cup veggie stock, low-sodium

Directions:
1. In slow cooker, combine the fennel with the lime juice, zest and the other ingredients, put the lid on and cook on Low for 2 hours and 30 minutes.
2. Divide between plates and serve as a side dish.

Nutrition: Calories 47, Fat 0.6g, Cholesterol 0mg, Sodium 71mg, Carbohydrate 10.8g, Fiber 4.3g, Sugars 0.4g, Protein 1.7g, Potassium 521mg

Butternut Mix

Preparation time: 10 minutes | Cooking time: 4 hours | Servings: 8

Ingredients:
- 1 cup carrots, chopped
- 1 tablespoon olive oil
- 1 yellow onion, chopped
- ½ teaspoon stevia
- 1 garlic clove, minced
- ½ teaspoon curry powder
- 1 butternut squash, cubed
- 2 and ½ cups low-sodium veggie stock
- ½ cup basmati rice
- ¾ cup coconut milk
- ½ teaspoon cinnamon powder
- ¼ teaspoon ginger, grated

Directions:
1. Heat up a pan with the oil over medium-high heat, add the oil, onion, garlic, stevia, carrots, curry powder, cinnamon and ginger, stir, cook for 5 minutes and transfer to your slow cooker.
2. Add squash, stock and coconut milk, stir, cover and cook on Low for 4 hours.
3. Divide the butternut mix between plates and serve as a side dish.

Nutrition: Calories 134, Fat 7.2g, Cholesterol 0mg, Sodium 59mg, Carbohydrate 16.5g, Fiber 1.7g, Sugars 2.7g, Protein 1.8g, Potassium 202mg

Sausage Side Dish

Preparation time: 10 minutes | Cooking time: 2 hours | Servings: 12

Ingredients:
- 6 celery ribs, chopped
- 1 pound no-sugar, beef sausage, chopped
- 2 tablespoons olive oil
- ½ pound mushrooms, chopped
- ½ cup sunflower seeds, peeled
- 1 cup low-sodium veggie stock
- 1 cup cranberries, dried
- 2 yellow onions, chopped
- 2 garlic cloves, minced
- 1 tablespoon sage, dried
- 1 whole wheat bread loaf, cubed

Directions:
1. Heat up a pan with the oil over medium-high heat, add beef, stir and brown for a few minutes.
2. Add mushrooms, onion, celery, garlic and sage, stir, cook for a few more minutes and transfer to your slow cooker.
3. Add stock, cranberries, sunflower seeds and the bread cubes, cover and cook on High for 2 hours.
4. Stir the whole mix, divide between plates and serve as a side dish.

Nutrition: Calories 188, Fat 13.8g, Cholesterol 25mg, Sodium 489mg, Carbohydrate 8.2g, Fiber 1.9g, Sugars 2.2g, Protein 7.6g, Potassium 254mg

Easy Potatoes Mix

Preparation time: 10 minutes | Cooking time: 6 hours | Servings: 8

Ingredients:
- 16 baby red potatoes, halved
- 2 cups low-sodium chicken stock
- 1 carrot, sliced
- 1 celery rib, chopped
- ¼ cup yellow onion, chopped
- 1 tablespoon parsley, chopped
- 2 tablespoons olive oil
- A pinch of black pepper
- 1 garlic clove minced

Directions:
1. In your slow cooker, mix the potatoes with the carrot, celery, onion, stock, parsley, garlic, oil and black pepper, toss, cover and cook on Low for 6 hours.
2. Divide between plates and serve as a side dish.

Nutrition: Calories 257, Fat 9.5g, Cholesterol 0mg, Sodium 845mg, Carbohydrate 43.4g, Fiber 4.4g, Sugars 4.6g, Protein 4.4g, Potassium 47mg

Black-Eyed Peas Mix

Preparation time: 10 minutes | Cooking time: 5 hours | Servings: 12

Ingredients:

- 17 ounces black-eyed peas
- 1 sweet red pepper, chopped
- ½ cup sausage, chopped
- 1 yellow onion, chopped
- 1 jalapeno, chopped
- 2 garlic cloves minced
- 6 cups water
- ½ teaspoon cumin, ground
- A pinch of black pepper
- 2 tablespoons cilantro, chopped

Directions:

1. In your slow cooker, mix the peas with the sausage, onion, red pepper, jalapeno, garlic, cumin, black pepper, water and cilantro, cover and cook on Low for 5 hours.
2. Divide between plates and serve as a side dish.

Nutrition: Calories 75, Fat 3.5g, Cholesterol 9mg, Sodium 94mg, Carbohydrate 7.2g, Fiber 1.7g, Sugars 0.9g, Protein 4.3g, Potassium 142mg

Green Beans and Corn Mix

Preparation time: 10 minutes | Cooking time: 4 hours | Servings: 8

Ingredients:

- 15 ounces green beans
- 14 ounces corn
- 4 ounces mushrooms, sliced
- 11 ounces cream of mushroom soup, low-fat and sodium-free
- ½ cup low-fat sour cream
- ½ cup almonds, chopped
- ½ cup low-fat cheddar cheese, shredded

Directions:

1. In your slow cooker, mix the green beans with the corn, mushrooms soup, mushrooms, almonds, cheese and sour cream, toss, cover and cook on Low for 4 hours.
2. Stir one more time, divide between plates and serve as a side dish.

Nutrition: Calories360, Fat 12.7g, Cholesterol 14mg, Sodium 220mg, Carbohydrate 58.3g, Fiber 10g, Sugars 10.3g, Protein 14g, Potassium 967mg

Minty Brussels Sprouts

Preparation time: 10 minutes | Cooking time: 3 hours | Servings: 4

Ingredients:

- 1 cup low-sodium veggie stock
- 1 pound Brussels sprouts, trimmed and halved
- 1 teaspoon rosemary, dried
- 1 teaspoon cumin, ground
- 1 tablespoon mint, chopped

Directions:

1. In your slow cooker, combine the sprouts with the stock and the other ingredients, put the lid on and cook on Low for 3 hours.
2. Divide between plates and serve as a side dish.

Nutrition: Calories 56, Fat 0.6g, Cholesterol 0mg, Sodium 65mg, Carbohydrate 11.4g, Fiber 4.5g, Sugars 2.7g, Protein 4g, Potassium 460mg

Spiced Carrots

Preparation time: 10 minutes | Cooking time: 6 hours | Servings: 6

Ingredients:

- 2 pounds small carrots, peeled
- ½ cup low-fat butter, melted
- ½ cup canned peach, unsweetened
- 2 tablespoons cornstarch
- 3 tablespoons stevia
- 2 tablespoons water
- ½ teaspoon cinnamon powder
- 1 teaspoon vanilla extract
- A pinch of nutmeg, ground

Directions:

1. In your slow cooker, mix the carrots with the butter, peach, stevia, cinnamon, vanilla, nutmeg and cornstarch mixed with water, toss, cover and cook on Low for 6 hours.
2. Toss the carrots one more time, divide between plates and serve as a side dish.

Nutrition: Calories139, Fat 10.7g, Cholesterol 0mg, Sodium 199mg, Carbohydrate 35.4g, Fiber 4.2g, Sugars 6.9g, Protein 3.8g, Potassium 25mg

Squash and Grains Mix

Preparation time: 10 minutes | Cooking time: 4 hours | Servings: 12

Ingredients:

- 1 butternut squash, peeled and cubed
- 1 cup whole grain blend, uncooked
- 12 ounces low-sodium veggie stock
- 6 ounces baby spinach
- 1 yellow onion, chopped
- 3 garlic cloves, minced
- ½ cup water
- 2 teaspoons thyme, chopped
- A pinch of black pepper

Directions:

1. In your slow cooker, mix the squash with the whole grain, onion, garlic, water, thyme, black pepper, stock and spinach, cover and
2. Divide between plates and serve as a side

dish.

Nutrition: Calories78, Fat 0.6g, Cholesterol 0mg, Sodium 259mg, Carbohydrate 16.4g, Fiber 1.8g, Sugars 2g, Protein 2.5g, Potassium 138mg

Mushroom Mix

Preparation time: 10 minutes | Cooking time: 4 hours | Servings: 6

Ingredients:

- 1 pound mushrooms, halved
- 1 teaspoon Italian seasoning
- 3 tablespoons olive oil
- 1 cup tomato sauce, no-salt-added
- 1 yellow onion, chopped

Directions:

1. In your slow cooker, mix the mushrooms with the oil, onion, Italian seasoning and tomato sauce, toss, cover and cook on Low for 4 hours.
2. Divide between plates and serve as a side dish.

Nutrition: Calories96, Fat 7.5g, Cholesterol 1mg, Sodium 219mg, Carbohydrate 6.5g, Fiber 1.8g, Sugars 3.9g, Protein 3.1g, Potassium 403mg

Spinach and Rice

Preparation time: 10 minutes | Cooking time: 4 hours | Servings: 8

Ingredients:

- 20 ounces spinach, chopped
- 8 ounces fat-free cream cheese
- 2 tablespoons olive oil
- 2 cups wild rice
- 2 cups low-fat cheddar cheese, shredded
- 1 yellow onion, chopped
- ¼ teaspoon thyme, dried
- 2 garlic cloves, minced
- 4 cups low-sodium chicken stock
- ½ cup whole wheat bread, crumbled

Directions:

1. In your slow cooker, mix the oil with the onion, thyme, garlic, stock, spinach, cream cheese and rice, toss, cover and cook on Low for 4 hours.
2. Add the cheese and the breadcrumbs, cover the pot, leave it aside for a few minutes, divide between plates and serve as a side dish.

Nutrition: Calories 448, Fat 24g, Cholesterol 61mg, Sodium 460mg, Carbohydrate 41.4g, Fiber 5.4g, Sugars 2.9g, Protein 19.7g, Potassium 688mg

Green Beans Salad

Preparation time: 40 minutes | Cooking time: 3 hours | Servings: 4

Ingredients:

- 1 pound green beans, trimmed and halved
- 2 teaspoons avocado oil
- 1 cup low-sodium veggie stock
- 2 garlic cloves, minced
- Zest of 1 lemon, grated
- 1 teaspoon hot paprika
- Juice of 1 lemon

Directions:

1. In your slow cooker, combine the green beans with the oil, stock and the other ingredients, put the lid on and cook on Low for 3 hours.
2. Divide between plates and serve as a side dish.

Nutrition: Calories 48, Fat 0.6g, Cholesterol 0mg, Sodium 77mg, Carbohydrate 9.6g, Fiber 4.1g, Sugars 2.2g, Protein 2.3g, Potassium 265mg

Creamy Mushrooms Mix

Preparation time: 10 minutes | Cooking time: 8 hours | Servings: 8

Ingredients:

- 1 and ½ pounds cremini mushrooms, halved
- ½ cup coconut cream
- 2 garlic cloves, minced
- 1 shallot, chopped
- ¼ cup low sodium chicken stock
- 2 tablespoons parsley, chopped
- 1 teaspoon cornstarch

Directions:

1. In your slow cooker, mix the mushrooms with garlic, shallot, stock and parsley, cover and cook on Low for 7 hours.
2. Add coconut cream mixed with the cornstarch, cover, cook on Low for 1 more hour, divide between plates and serve as a side dish.

Nutrition: Calories 62, Fat 3.7g, Cholesterol 0mg, Sodium 10mg, Carbohydrate 5.2g, Fiber 0.9g, Sugars 2g, Protein 2.6g, Potassium 433mg

Ginger Beets

Preparation time: 10 minutes | Cooking time: 6 hours | Servings: 8

Ingredients:

- 6 beets, peeled and sliced
- 1/3 cup orange juice
- 1 teaspoon orange peel, grated
- 2 tablespoons stevia
- 1 tablespoon ginger, grated
- A pinch of black pepper
- 2 tablespoons white vinegar

- 2 tablespoons olive oil

Directions:
1. In your slow cooker, mix the beets with the orange peel, orange juice, stevia, vinegar, oil, ginger and black pepper, toss, cover and cook on Low for 6 hours.
2. Divide between plates and serve as a side dish.

Nutrition: Calories 71, Fat 3.7g, Cholesterol 0mg, Sodium 58mg, Carbohydrate 12.9g, Fiber 1.6g, Sugars 6.9g, Protein 1.4g, Potassium 262mg

Artichokes Mix

Preparation time: 10 minutes | Cooking time: 5 hours | Servings: 8

Ingredients:
- 4 artichokes, trimmed and halved
- 2 cups whole wheat breadcrumbs
- 1 cup low-sodium vegetable stock
- Juice of 1 lemon
- 3 garlic cloves, minced
- 1 tablespoon lemon zest, grated
- 2 tablespoons parsley, chopped
- 1/3 cup low-fat parmesan, grated
- Black pepper to the taste
- 1 tablespoon olive oil
- 1 tablespoon shallot, minced
- 1 teaspoon oregano, chopped

Directions:
1. Rub artichokes with the lemon juice and the oil and put them in your slow cooker.
2. Add breadcrumbs, garlic, parsley, parmesan, lemon zest, black pepper, shallot, oregano and stock, cover and cook on Low for 5 hours.
3. Divide the whole mix between plates, sprinkle parsley on top and serve as a side dish.

Nutrition: Calories 149, Fat 2.8g, Cholesterol 1mg, Sodium 188mg, Carbohydrate 26g, Fiber 6.7g, Sugars 2.1g, Protein 7.7g, Potassium 368mg

Creamy Corn

Preparation time: 10 minutes | Cooking time: 2 hours | Servings: 6

Ingredients:
- 3 cups corn
- 1 cup low-sodium veggie stock
- ½ teaspoon cayenne pepper
- ½ teaspoon turmeric powder
- ½ teaspoon nutmeg, ground
- ¼ cup coconut cream
- Black pepper to the taste
- 1 tablespoon dill, chopped

Directions:
1. In your slow cooker, combine the corn with the stock, cayenne and the other ingredients, put the lid on and cook on High for 2 hours.
2. Divide the mix between plates and serve as a side dish.

Nutrition: Calories 117, Fat 4.4g, Cholesterol 0mg, Sodium 266mg, Carbohydrate 19.1g, Fiber 2.6 g, Sugars 4.6g, Protein 3g, Potassium 260mg

Asparagus Mix

Preparation time: 10 minutes | Cooking time: 2 hours | Servings: 4

Ingredients:
- 1 pound asparagus, trimmed and halved
- 1 tablespoon parsley, chopped
- ¼ teaspoon lemon zest, grated
- 2 teaspoons lemon juice
- ½ cup low-sodium veggie stock
- 1 garlic clove, minced

Directions:
1. In your slow cooker, mix the asparagus with the parsley, stock, garlic, lemon zest and lemon juice, toss a bit, cover and cook on High for 2 hours.
2. Divide the asparagus between plates and serve as a side dish.

Nutrition: Calories 27, Fat 0.2g, Cholesterol 0mg, Sodium 21mg, Carbohydrate 5g, Fiber 2.5g, Sugars 2.3g, Protein 2.6g, Potassium 241mg

Black Bean and Corn Mix

Preparation time: 10 minutes | Cooking time: 6 hours | Servings: 6

Ingredients:
- 16 ounces canned black beans, drained
- 4 tomatoes, chopped
- 1 cup corn kernels
- 1 small red onion, chopped
- 1 red bell pepper, chopped
- 2 garlic cloves, minced
- ½ cup parsley, chopped
- Juice of 1 lemon
- 2 tablespoons stevia

Directions:
1. In your slow cooker, mix the tomatoes with corn, black beans, garlic, parsley, lemon juice, bell pepper, onion and stevia, toss, cook on Low for 6 hours, divide between plates and serve as a side dish.

Nutrition: Calories 311, Fat 1.7g, Cholesterol 0mg, Sodium 17mg, Carbohydrate 62.7g, Fiber 13.9g, Sugars 6.3g, Protein 18.5g, Potassium 1481mg

Celery Mix

Preparation time: 10 minutes | Cooking time: 3 hours | Servings: 3

Ingredients:

- 2 celery roots, cut into medium wedges
- ¼ cup low-fat sour cream
- 1 cup low-sodium veggie stock
- 1 teaspoon mustard
- 2 teaspoons thyme, chopped
- Black pepper to the taste

Directions:

1. In your slow cooker, mix the celery with the stock, mustard, cream, black pepper and thyme, cover and cook on High for 3 hours.
2. Divide the celery between plates, drizzle some of the cooking juices on top and serve as a side dish.

Nutrition: Calories 103, Fat 5g, Cholesterol 8mg, Sodium 217mg, Carbohydrate 12.7g, Fiber 2.3g, Sugars 2.6g, Protein 2.6g, Potassium 353mg

Kale Side Dish

Preparation time: 10 minutes | Cooking time: 2 hours | Servings: 6

Ingredients:

- 1 pound kale, chopped
- 2 teaspoons olive oil
- 1 tablespoons lemon juice
- 4 garlic cloves, minced
- ½ cup low-sodium veggie stock
- 1 cup cherry tomatoes, halved
- Black pepper to the taste

Directions:

1. Heat up a pan with the oil over medium heat, add garlic, stir, cook for 2 minutes and transfer to your slow cooker.
2. Add kale, stock, tomatoes, black pepper and lemon juice, cover, cook on High for 2 hours.
3. Divide the whole mix between plates and serve as a side dish.

Nutrition: Calories 65, Fat 1.9g, Cholesterol 8mg, Sodium 84mg, Carbohydrate 10.5g, Fiber 1.6g, Sugars 1.2g, Protein 2.7g, Potassium 453mg

Spicy Eggplant

Preparation time: 10 minutes | Cooking time: 3 hours | Servings: 4

Ingredients:

- 2 cups cherry tomatoes, halved
- 1 eggplant, sliced
- ½ teaspoon cumin, ground
- A pinch of nutmeg, ground
- ½ yellow onion, chopped
- 1 tablespoon cilantro, chopped
- 1 teaspoon mustard seed
- ½ teaspoon coriander, ground
- ½ teaspoon curry powder
- 1 teaspoon red wine vinegar
- 1 tablespoon olive oil
- 1 garlic clove, minced
- Black pepper to the taste

Directions:

1. Grease the slow cooker with the oil and add eggplant slices inside.
2. Add cumin, mustard seeds, coriander, curry powder, nutmeg, tomatoes, onion, garlic, vinegar, black pepper and cilantro, cover and cook on High for 3 hours.
3. Divide between plates and serve as a side dish.

Nutrition: Calories 94, Fat 4.6g, Cholesterol 0mg, Sodium 64mg, Carbohydrate 13.2g, Fiber 5.7g, Sugars 7g, Protein 2.5g, Potassium 514mg

Corn Salad

Preparation time: 10 minutes | Cooking time: 2 hours | Servings: 6

Ingredients:

- 2 ounces prosciutto, cut into strips
- 1 teaspoon olive oil
- 2 cups corn
- ½ cup salt-free tomato sauce
- 1 green bell pepper, chopped
- 1 teaspoon garlic, minced

Directions:

1. Grease your slow cooker with the oil, add corn, prosciutto, tomato sauce, garlic and bell pepper, cover and cook on High for 2 hours.
2. Divide between plates and serve as a side dish.

Nutrition: Calories 79, Fat 1.9g, Cholesterol 5mg, Sodium 130mg, Carbohydrate 13.5g, Fiber 2.1g, Sugars 3.9g, Protein 4.2g, Potassium 274mg

Spinach and Sprouts Salad

Preparation time: 10 minutes | Cooking time: 2 hours | Servings: 4

Ingredients:

- 1 pound baby spinach
- ½ pound Brussels sprouts, trimmed and halved
- 2 teaspoons avocado oil
- 1 red onion, sliced
- ½ teaspoon chili powder
- 2 tomatoes, cubed
- ½ cup low sodium veggie stock
- Black pepper to the taste

Directions:

1. In your slow cooker, combine the spinach

with the sprouts, oil and the other ingredients, put the lid on and cook on High for 2 hours.
2. Divide the mix between plates and serve as a side dish.

Nutrition: Calories 111, Fat 2.6g, Cholesterol 0mg, Sodium 440mg, Carbohydrate 19.3g, Fiber 6.3g, Sugars 6.9g, Protein 6.3g, Potassium 1053mg

Spiced Cabbage

Preparation time: 10 minutes | Cooking time: 4 hours | Servings: 6

Ingredients:
- 2 yellow onions, chopped
- 10 cups red cabbage, shredded
- 1 cup plums, pitted and chopped
- 1 teaspoon cinnamon powder
- 1 garlic clove, minced
- 1 teaspoon cumin seeds
- 1 teaspoon coriander seeds
- ¼ teaspoon cloves, ground
- 2 tablespoons red wine vinegar
- ½ cup water

Directions:
1. In your slow cooker, mix cabbage with onions, plums, garlic, cinnamon, cumin, cloves, vinegar, coriander and water, stir, cover and cook on Low for 4 hours.
2. Divide between plates and serve as a side dish.

Nutrition: Calories 52, Fat 0.3g, Cholesterol 0mg, Sodium 24mg, Carbohydrate 12g, Fiber 3.9g, Sugars 6.5g, Protein 2.1g, Potassium 283mg

Spinach and Beans Mix

Preparation time: 10 minutes | Cooking time: 4 hours | Servings: 6

Ingredients:
- 5 carrots, sliced
- 5 ounces baby spinach
- 1 yellow onion, chopped
- 1 and ½ cups great northern beans, dried
- 2 garlic cloves, minced
- 2 teaspoons lemon peel, grated
- 3 tablespoons lemon juice
- Black pepper to the taste
- ½ teaspoon oregano, dried
- 4 and ½ cups low-sodium veggie stock

Directions:
1. In your slow cooker, mix beans with onion, carrots, garlic, pepper, oregano and stock, stir, cover and cook on High for 4 hours.
2. Add spinach, lemon juice and lemon peel, stir, leave aside for 5 minutes, divide between plates and serve.

Nutrition: Calories 208, Fat 0.9g, Cholesterol 0mg, Sodium 152mg, Carbohydrate 38.1g, Fiber 11.6g, Sugars 4.9g, Protein 13g, Potassium 973mg

Sage Sweet Potatoes

Preparation time: 10 minutes | Cooking time: 3 hours | Servings: 10

Ingredients:
- 4 pounds sweet potatoes, sliced
- 3 tablespoons stevia
- 2 tablespoons olive oil
- ½ teaspoon sage, dried
- ½ cup orange juice
- ½ teaspoon thyme, dried
- A pinch of black pepper

Directions:
1. In a bowl, mix orange juice with salt, pepper, stevia, thyme, sage and oil and whisk well.
2. Add the potatoes to your slow cooker, drizzle the sage and orange mix all over, cover, cook on High for 3 hours, divide between plates and serve as a side dish.

Nutrition: Calories 244, Fat 0.3g, Cholesterol 0mg, Sodium 16mg, Carbohydrate 56.4g, Fiber 7.5g, Sugars 2g, Protein 2.9g, Potassium 1506mg

Garlicky Potato Mash

Preparation time: 10 minutes | Cooking time: 4 hours | Servings: 6

Ingredients:
- 3 pounds gold potatoes, peeled and cubed
- 6 garlic cloves, peeled
- 28 ounces low-sodium veggie stock
- 1 bay leaf
- 1 cup coconut milk
- 3 tablespoons olive oil
- Black pepper to the taste

Directions:
1. In your slow cooker, mix potatoes with stock, bay leaf, garlic, salt and pepper, cover and cook on High for 4 hours.
2. Drain potatoes and garlic, mash them, add oil and milk, whisk well, divide between plates and serve as a side dish.

Nutrition: Calories 321, Fat 16.8g, Cholesterol 0mg, Sodium 121mg, Carbohydrate 41.2g, Fiber 7g, Sugars 5.2g, Protein 4.2g, Potassium 1055mg

Creamy Cauliflower

Preparation time: 10 minutes | Cooking time: 4 hours | Servings: 4

Ingredients:
- 1 pound cauliflower florets

- 2 teaspoons avocado oil
- 1 cup coconut cream
- ½ teaspoon garam masala
- 3 garlic cloves, minced
- ½ teaspoon ginger, ground
- Black pepper to the taste
- ¼ cup chives, chopped

Directions:
1. In your slow cooker, combine the cauliflower with the oil, cream and the other ingredients, put the lid on and cook on Low for 4 hours.
2. Divide between plates and serve as a side dish.

Nutrition: Calories 207, Fat 16.3g, Cholesterol 0mg, Sodium 324mg, Carbohydrate 14.7g, Fiber 4.6g, Sugars 7.1g, Protein 4.2g, Potassium 530mg

Chickpeas Side Dish

Preparation time: 10 minutes | Cooking time: 8 hours | Servings: 6

Ingredients:
- 30 ounces canned chickpeas, no-salt-added, drained and rinsed
- 28 ounces low-sodium veggie stock
- 4 cups baby spinach
- 8 ounces zucchini, sliced
- A pinch of black pepper
- 2 cups cherry tomatoes, halved
- 2 garlic cloves, minced
- 1 cup corn
- 7 small baby carrots
- 2 tablespoons olive oil
- 2 tablespoons rosemary, chopped

Directions:
1. In your slow cooker, mix chickpeas with oil, rosemary, pepper, cherry tomatoes, garlic, corn, baby carrots, zucchini, spinach and stock, stir, cover, cook on Low for 8 hours, divide between plates and serve.

Nutrition: Calories 617, Fat 14g, Cholesterol 0mg, Sodium 147mg, Carbohydrate 98.2g, Fiber 27.8g, Sugars 19.4g, Protein 29.9g, Potassium 1705mg

Warm Eggplant Salad

Preparation time: 10 minutes | Cooking time: 2 hours | Servings: 6

Ingredients:
- 14 ounces canned roasted tomatoes, no-salt-added and chopped
- 4 cups kale, torn
- 4 cups eggplant, cubed
- 1 yellow bell pepper, chopped
- 1 red onion, cut into medium wedges
- 3 tablespoons red vinegar
- 1 garlic clove, minced
- 2 tablespoons olive oil
- 1 teaspoon mustard
- ½ cup parsley, chopped
- A pinch of black pepper

Directions:
1. In your slow cooker, mix eggplant with tomatoes, bell pepper and onion, cover and cook on High for 2 hours.
2. In a bowl, mix oil with vinegar, mustard, garlic and pepper, whisk well, add to your slow cooker, also add kale and parsley, toss, divide between plates and serve as a side dish.

Nutrition: Calories 103, Fat 5g, Cholesterol 0mg, Sodium 175mg, Carbohydrate 14.8g, Fiber 4.2g, Sugars 4.3g, Protein 2.9g, Potassium 556mg

Garlic and Rosemary Potato Mix

Preparation time: 10 minutes | Cooking time: 3 hours | Servings: 12

Ingredients:
- 3 pounds baby potatoes, halved
- 7 garlic cloves, minced
- 2 tablespoons olive oil
- 1 tablespoon rosemary, chopped
- A pinch of black pepper

Directions:
1. In your slow cooker, mix oil with potatoes, garlic, rosemary and pepper, toss, cover, cook on High for 3 hours, divide between plates and serve.

Nutrition: Calories 89, Fat 2.5g, Cholesterol 0mg, Sodium 12mg, Carbohydrate 14.9g, Fiber 3g, Sugars 0g, Protein 3g, Potassium 478mg

Apple Brussels sprouts

Preparation time: 10 minutes | Cooking time: 3 hours | Servings: 12

Ingredients:
- 1 cup red onion, chopped
- ¼ cup natural apple juice, unsweetened
- 2 pounds Brussels sprouts, trimmed and halved
- 3 tablespoons olive oil
- 1 tablespoon cilantro, chopped
- A pinch of black pepper

Directions:
1. In your slow cooker, mix Brussels sprouts with onion, oil, cilantro, pepper and apple juice, toss, cover and cook on Low for 3 hours.
2. Toss well, divide between plates and serve as a side dish.

Nutrition: Calories 69, Fat 3.8g, Cholesterol 0mg, Sodium 20mg, Carbohydrate 8.4g, Fiber 3.1g, Sugars 2.7g, Protein 2.7g, Potassium 312mg

Tomato Salad

Preparation time: 10 minutes | Cooking time: 3 hours | Servings: 4

Ingredients:
- 1 pound tomatoes, cut into wedges
- 1 tablespoon olive oil
- ½ teaspoon garlic powder
- ½ teaspoon sweet paprika
- ½ teaspoon chili powder
- ½ teaspoon onion powder
- 1 cup low-sodium veggie stock
- 2 tablespoons oregano, chopped

Directions:
1. In the slow cooker, combine the tomatoes with the oil, garlic powder and the other ingredients, put the lid on and cook on Low for 3 hours.
2. Divide the mix between plates and serve as a side dish.

Nutrition: Calories 65, Fat 4.1g, Cholesterol 0mg, Sodium 107mg, Carbohydrate 7.7g, Fiber 2.6g, Sugars 3.6g, Protein 1.4g, Potassium 325mg

Italian Beans Mix

Preparation time: 10 minutes | Cooking time: 6 hours | Servings: 8

Ingredients:
- 38 ounces canned cannellini beans, no-salt-added, drained and rinsed
- 19 ounces canned fava beans, no-salt-added, drained and rinsed
- 1 yellow onion, chopped
- 3 tomatoes, chopped
- 2 cups spinach
- 1 cup radicchio, torn
- ¼ cup basil, chopped
- 4 garlic cloves, minced
- 1 and ½ teaspoon Italian seasoning
- 1 tablespoon olive oil

Directions:
1. In your slow cooker, mix cannellini beans with fava beans, oil, basil, onion, garlic, Italian seasoning, tomato, spinach and radicchio, toss, cover, cook on Low for 6 hours, divide between plates and serve as a side dish.

Nutrition: Calories 715, Fat 4.3g, Cholesterol 1mg, Sodium 51mg, Carbohydrate 124.2g, Fiber 51.5g, Sugars 8.8g, Protein 50.3g, Potassium 2803mg

Tomatoes, Okra and Zucchini Mix

Preparation time: 10 minutes | Cooking time: 3 hours | Servings: 4

Ingredients:
- 1 cup cherry tomatoes, halved
- 1 and ½ cups red onion, cut into wedges
- 2 cups okra, sliced
- 2 cups yellow bell pepper, chopped
- 1 cup mushrooms, sliced
- 2 and ½ cups zucchini, sliced
- 1 tablespoon thyme, chopped
- 2 tablespoons basil, chopped
- ½ cup olive oil
- ½ cup balsamic vinegar

Directions:
1. In a large bowl, mix onion with tomatoes, okra, zucchini, bell pepper, mushrooms, basil, thyme, oil and vinegar, cover and cook on High for 3 hours.
2. Divide between plates and serve as a side dish.

Nutrition: Calories 304, Fat 25.8g, Cholesterol 0mg, Sodium 19mg, Carbohydrate 17.7g, Fiber 5.1g, Sugars 8.4g, Protein 3.9g, Potassium 703mg

Easy Cabbage

Preparation time: 10 minutes | Cooking time: 6 hours | Servings: 4

Ingredients:
- 1 onion, sliced
- 1 cabbage, shredded
- 2 apples, peeled, cored and roughly chopped
- 3 tablespoons mustard
- 1 tablespoon olive oil
- 1 cup low-sodium chicken stock
- Black pepper to the taste

Directions:
1. Grease your slow cooker with the oil and add apples, cabbage and onions.
2. In a bowl, mix stock with mustard and black pepper, whisk well, pour this into your slow cooker, cover, cook on Low for 6 hours, divide between plates and serve as a side dish.

Nutrition: Calories 148, Fat 6.5g, Cholesterol 0mg, Sodium 93mg, Carbohydrate 22.1g, Fiber 4.7g, Sugars 14g, Protein 3.1g, Potassium 227mg

Acorn Squash Mix

Preparation time: 10 minutes | Cooking time: 7 hours | Servings: 4

Ingredients:
- 16 ounces canned cranberry sauce, unsweetened
- 2 acorn squash, peeled and cut into medium wedges

- ¼ teaspoon cinnamon powder
- Black pepper to the taste

Directions:
1. Put the acorn wedges in your slow cooker; add cranberry sauce, raisins, cinnamon and pepper, stir, cover, cook on Low for 7 hours, divide between plates and serve.

Nutrition: Calories 155, Fat 0.5g, Cholesterol 0mg, Sodium 62mg, Carbohydrate 33.6g, Fiber 7.4g, Sugars 4.6g, Protein 1.8g, Potassium 941mg

Spring Onions and Peas Mix

Preparation time: 10 minutes | Cooking time: 2 hours | Servings: 4

Ingredients:
- 1 red onion, sliced
- ½ cup spring onions, chopped
- 1 pound green peas
- 1 tablespoon avocado oil
- 1 teaspoon coriander, ground
- ½ teaspoon rosemary, dried
- 4 water low-sodium veggie stock
- A pinch of black pepper

Directions:
1. In your slow cooker, combine the onion with the peas, spring onions and the other ingredients, put the lid on and cook on High for 2 hours..
2. Divide the mix between plates and serve as a side dish.

Nutrition: Calories 127, Fat 1g, Cholesterol 0mg, Sodium 149mg, Carbohydrate 22.2g, Fiber 6.9g, Sugars 8.9g, Protein 6.7g, Potassium 365mg

Italian Zucchini and Squash

Preparation time: 10 minutes | Cooking time: 6 hours | Servings: 6

Ingredients:
- 2 cups zucchinis, sliced
- 1 teaspoon Italian seasoning
- 1 teaspoon garlic powder
- 2 tablespoons olive oil
- 2 cups yellow squash, peeled and cut into wedges
- Black pepper to the taste

Directions:
1. Grease the slow cooker with the oil, add zucchini, squash, Italian seasoning, black pepper and garlic powder, toss well, cover, cook on Low for 6 hours, divide between plates and serve as a side dish.

Nutrition: Calories 61, Fat 5.2g, Cholesterol 1mg, Sodium 51mg, Carbohydrate 3.7g, Fiber 1.1g, Sugars 1.7g, Protein 1g, Potassium 104mg

Coconut Broccoli

Preparation time: 10 minutes | Cooking time: 3 hours | Servings: 10

Ingredients:
- 10 ounces coconut cream
- 6 cups broccoli florets, chopped
- 1 and ½ cups low-fat cheese, shredded
- 2 tablespoons olive oil
- ¼ cup yellow onion, chopped

Directions:
1. Add the oil to your slow cooker, add broccoli, onion, coconut cream, sprinkle cheese, cover and cook on High for 3 hours.
2. Divide between plates and serve as a side dish.

Nutrition: Calories 177, Fat 15.4g, Cholesterol 18mg, Sodium 128mg, Carbohydrate 5.7g, Fiber 2.1g, Sugars 2.1g, Protein 6.4g, Potassium 268mg

Asian Green Beans

Preparation time: 10 minutes | Cooking time: 2 hours | Servings: 10

Ingredients:
- 16 cups green beans, halved
- ½ cup coconut sugar
- ¼ cup tomato sauce, no-salt-added
- ¾ teaspoon low sodium soy sauce
- 3 tablespoons olive oil
- A pinch of black pepper

Directions:
1. In your slow cooker, mix green beans with coconut sugar, tomato sauce, pepper, soy sauce and oil, cover and cook on Low for 3 hours.
2. Divide between plates and serve as a side dish.

Nutrition: Calories 98, Fat 4.4g, Cholesterol 0mg, Sodium 58mg, Carbohydrate 13.9g, Fiber 6.1g, Sugars 2.7g, Protein 3.4g, Potassium 389mg

Cauliflower Rice and Mushrooms

Preparation time: 10 minutes | Cooking time: 3 hours | Servings: 6

Ingredients:
- ½ pound Portobello mushrooms, sliced
- 1 cup cauliflower, riced
- 6 green onions, chopped
- 2 cups water
- 2 garlic cloves, minced
- 3 tablespoons olive oil
- A pinch of black pepper

Directions:

1. In your slow cooker, mix cauliflower with green onions, oil, garlic, mushrooms, water and pepper, stir well, cover, cook on Low for 3 hours, divide between plates and serve as a side dish.

Nutrition: Calories 81, Fat 7.1g, Cholesterol 0mg, Sodium 10mg, Carbohydrate 3.4g, Fiber 0.8g, Sugars 0.8g, Protein 1.7g, Potassium 237mg

Cranberries, Cauliflower and Mushroom Mix

Preparation time: 10 minutes | Cooking time: 2 hours and 30 minutes | Servings: 12

Ingredients:
- 1 pound mushrooms, sliced
- 1 cup cranberries, dried
- 6 celery ribs, chopped
- 1 cup cauliflower florets, chopped
- 1 cup low-sodium veggie stock
- 2 yellow onions, chopped
- 2 garlic cloves, minced
- 1 tablespoon sage, chopped
- 1 tablespoons olive oil

Directions:
1. Add the oil to your slow cooker, add mushrooms, celery, onion, garlic, sage, cranberries, cauliflower and stock, stir, cover and cook on High for 2 hours and 30 minutes.
2. Divide between plates and serve as a side dish.

Nutrition: Calories 46, Fat 1.6g, Cholesterol 0mg, Sodium 40mg, Carbohydrate 6.3g, Fiber 2g, Sugars 2.8g, Protein 2.1g, Potassium 292mg

Creamy Cauliflower Rice

Preparation time: 10 minutes | Cooking time: 3 hours | Servings: 8

Ingredients:
- 3 cups low-sodium veggie stock
- 20 ounces spinach, chopped
- 2 garlic cloves, minced
- 6 ounces coconut cream
- 2 cups cauliflower rice
- 1 yellow onion, chopped
- ¼ teaspoon thyme, dried
- A pinch of black pepper
- 2 tablespoons olive oil

Directions:
1. Heat up a pan with the oil over medium heat, add onion, garlic, thyme and stock, stir, cook for 5 minutes and transfer to your slow cooker.
2. Add spinach, coconut cream, cauliflower rice and pepper, cover, cook on High for 3 hours, divide between plates and serve as a side dish.

Nutrition: Calories 122, Fat 9.3g, Cholesterol 0mg, Sodium 116mg, Carbohydrate 7.4g, Fiber 2.4g, Sugars 2.6g, Protein 4.5g, Potassium 475mg

Curry Zucchini Mix

Preparation time: 10 minutes | Cooking time: 3 hours | Servings: 4

Ingredients:
- 1 pound eggplants, roughly cubed
- 1 teaspoon fennel seeds, crushed
- ½ teaspoon rosemary, dried
- 2 tablespoons red curry paste
- ½ teaspoon curry powder
- 1 tablespoon olive oil
- 1 garlic clove, minced
- A pinch of black pepper
- 1 and ½ cups coconut cream
- 1 tablespoon parsley, chopped

Directions:
1. In the slow cooker, combine the eggplants with the crushed fennel rosemary and the other ingredients, put the lid on and cook on Low for 3 hours.
2. Divide the eggplant mix between plates and serve.

Nutrition: Calories 300, Fat 27.5g, Cholesterol 0mg, Sodium 407mg, Carbohydrate 14g, Fiber 6.4g, Sugars 6.4g, Protein 3.4g, Potassium 519mg

Creamy and Cheesy Spinach

Preparation time: 10 minutes | Cooking time: 5 hours | Servings: 6

Ingredients:
- 1 cup low-fat cheese, shredded
- 2 cups coconut cream
- 20 ounces spinach
- 2 tablespoons olive oil

Directions:
1. In your slow cooker, mix spinach with coconut cream, oil and cheese, cover and cook on Low for 5 hours.
2. Divide between plates and serve as a side dish.

Nutrition: Calories 322, Fat 30.4g, Cholesterol 20mg, Sodium 204mg, Carbohydrate 8.1g, Fiber 3.8g, Sugars 3.2g, Protein 9.2g, Potassium 756mg

Dill Cauliflower Mash

Preparation time: 10 minutes | Cooking time: 5 hours | Servings: 6

Ingredients:

- 1/3 cup dill, chopped
- 1 cauliflower head, florets separated
- 6 garlic cloves
- A pinch of black pepper
- 2 tablespoons olive oil

Directions:
1. Put cauliflower in your slow cooker, add dill, garlic and water to cover them, cover, cook on High for 5 hours, drain, add pepper and oil, mash using a potato masher, whisk well and serve as a side dish.

Nutrition: Calories 62, Fat 4.9g, Cholesterol 0mg, Sodium 19mg, Carbohydrate 4.8g, Fiber 1.5g, Sugars 1.1g, Protein 1.6g, Potassium 234mg

Baby Spinach and Avocado Mix

Preparation time: 10 minutes | Cooking time: 4 hours | Servings: 6

Ingredients:
- 5 carrots, sliced
- 5 ounces baby spinach
- 1 avocado, pitted, peeled and chopped
- 1 yellow onion, chopped
- A pinch of black pepper
- 2 garlic cloves, minced
- ½ teaspoon oregano, dried
- 2 and ½ cups low-sodium veggie stock
- 2 teaspoons lemon peel, grated
- 3 tablespoons lemon juice

Directions:
1. In your slow cooker, mix onion, carrots, garlic, pepper, oregano and stock, stir, cover and cook on High for 4 hours.
2. Add spinach, lemon juice and lemon peel, stir, leave aside for 5 minutes, divide between plates, sprinkle avocado on top and serve as a side dish.

Nutrition: Calories 112, Fat 6.7g, Cholesterol 0mg, Sodium 116mg, Carbohydrate 12g, Fiber 4.7g, Sugars 4.2g, Protein 2.1g, Potassium 501mg

Simple Parsnips Mix

Preparation time: 10 minutes | Cooking time: 4 hours | Servings: 10

Ingredients:
- 3 pounds parsnips, cut into medium chunks
- 1 cup low-sodium veggie stock
- 2 tablespoons lemon peel, grated
- 3 tablespoons olive oil
- ¼ cup cilantro, chopped
- A pinch of black pepper

Directions:
1. In your slow cooker, mix parsnips with lemon peel, stock, pepper, oil and cilantro, cover, cook on High for 4 hours, divide between plates and serve as a side dish.

Nutrition: Calories 140, Fat 4.6g, Cholesterol 0mg, Sodium 21mg, Carbohydrate 24.9g, Fiber 6.8g, Sugars 6.6g, Protein 1.9g, Potassium 516mg

Basil and Oregano Mushrooms

Preparation time: 10 minutes | Cooking time: 4 hours | Servings: 4

Ingredients:
- 4 garlic cloves, minced
- 24 ounces white mushrooms, halved
- 1 teaspoon basil, dried
- 1 teaspoon oregano, dried
- 2 tablespoons olive oil
- 2 tablespoons parsley, chopped
- ¼ teaspoon thyme dried
- 1 cup low-sodium veggie stock
- A pinch of black pepper

Directions:
1. Grease the slow cooker with the oil, add mushrooms, garlic, bay leaves, thyme, basil, oregano, black pepper, parsley and stock, cover, cook on Low for 4 hours, divide between plates and serve as a side dish.

Nutrition: Calories 108, Fat 7.6g, Cholesterol 0mg, Sodium 46mg, Carbohydrate 7.5g, Fiber 2g, Sugars 3.2g, Protein 5.7g, Potassium 571mg

Minty Okra

Preparation time: 10 minutes | Cooking time: 3 hours | Servings: 4

Ingredients:
- 1 pound okra, sliced
- 2 tablespoons mint, chopped
- 2 teaspoons olive oil
- 4 green onions, chopped
- 2 tablespoons low-sodium chicken stock
- Black pepper to the taste

Directions:
1. Grease your slow cooker with the oil, add okra, pepper, mint, stock and green onions, toss, cover, cook on Low for 3 hours, divide between plates and serve as a side dish.

Nutrition: Calories 78, Fat 2.9g, Cholesterol 0mg, Sodium 71mg, Carbohydrate 10.6g, Fiber 4.2g, Sugars 2.5g, Protein 2.6g, Potassium 394mg

Cabbage, Radish and Carrot Mix

Preparation time: 10 minutes | Cooking time: 2 hours | Servings: 6

Ingredients:

- 1 pound green cabbage, chopped
- 3 green onion stalks, chopped
- 3 carrots, julienned
- 1 cup radish, sliced
- 3 tablespoons chili flakes
- 1 tablespoon olive oil
- ¼ cup low sodium veggie stock
- ½ pinch ginger, grated
- A pinch of black pepper

Directions:
1. In your slow cooker, mix cabbage with pepper, carrots, stock, radish, green onions, chili flakes, oil and ginger, toss, cover, cook on High for 2 hours, divide between plates and serve as a side dish.

Nutrition: Calories 65, Fat 2.5g, Cholesterol 0mg, Sodium 50mg, Carbohydrate 9.1g, Fiber 3.3g, Sugars 4.6g, Protein 1.6g, Potassium 304mg

Simple Swiss Chard Mix

Preparation time: 10 minutes | Cooking time: 2 hours | Servings: 4

Ingredients:
- 2 tablespoons olive oil
- 2 bunches Swiss chard, roughly torn
- 3 tablespoons lemon juice
- ½ cup low-sodium veggie stock
- Black pepper to the taste
- ½ teaspoon garlic paste

Directions:
1. In your slow cooker, mix oil with chard, stock, lemon juice, garlic paste and pepper, toss, cover, cook on High for 2 hours, divide between plates and serve.

Nutrition: Calories 75, Fat 7.4g, Cholesterol 0mg, Sodium 106mg, Carbohydrate 2g, Fiber 0.4g, Sugars 0.9g, Protein 0.7g, Potassium 84mg

Dash Diet Slow Cooker Snack and Appetizer Recipes

Eggplant Salsa

Preparation time: 10 minutes | Cooking time: 7 hours | Servings: 4

Ingredients:
- 3 cups eggplant, cubed
- 4 garlic cloves, minced
- 6 ounces green olives, pitted and sliced
- 1 and ½ cups tomatoes, chopped
- 2 teaspoons balsamic vinegar
- 1 tablespoon oregano, chopped
- Black pepper to the taste

Directions:
1. In your slow cooker, mix tomatoes with eggplant, green olives, garlic, vinegar, oregano and pepper, toss, cover, cook on Low for 7 hours, divide into small bowls and serve as an appetizer.

Nutrition: Calories 78, Fat 3.6g, Cholesterol 0mg, Sodium 443mg, Carbohydrate 11.2g, Fiber 4.6g, Sugars 4.2g, Protein 2g, Potassium 337mg

Zucchini Dip

Preparation time: 10 minutes | Cooking time: 2 hours | Servings: 4

Ingredients:
- 1 pound zucchinis, grated
- ½ cup coconut cream
- 1 teaspoon turmeric powder
- 8 ounces fat-free cream cheese
- 2 tablespoons chives, chopped
- 1 tablespoon dill, chopped

Directions:
1. In your slow cooker, combine the zucchinis with the cream, turmeric and the other ingredients, put the lid on and cook on Low for 2 hours.
2. Divide into bowls and serve as a party dip.

Nutrition: Calories 289, Fat 27.2g, Cholesterol 62mg, Sodium 186mg, Carbohydrate 7.8g, Fiber 2.2g, Sugars 3.1g, Protein 6.6g, Potassium 488mg

Artichoke and Beans Spread

Preparation time: 10 minutes | Cooking time: 30 minutes | Servings: 8

Ingredients:
- 4 cups spinach, chopped
- 2 cups artichoke hearts
- 1 cup white beans, already cooked
- 1 teaspoon thyme, chopped
- 2 garlic cloves, minced
- 1 tablespoon parsley, chopped
- 2 tablespoons low-fat parmesan, grated
- ½ cup low-fat sour cream
- Black pepper to the taste

Directions:
1. In your slow cooker, mix artichokes with spinach, black pepper, thyme, garlic, beans, parmesan, parsley and sour cream, stir, cover and cook on Low for 5 hours.
2. Transfer to your blender, pulse well divide into bowls and serve.

Nutrition: Calories 145, Fat 3.5g, Cholesterol 6mg, Sodium 123mg, Carbohydrate 21.9g, Fiber 6.5g, Sugars 1.3g, Protein 8.5g, Potassium 714mg

Stuffed White Mushrooms

Preparation time: 10 minutes | Cooking time: 5 hours | Servings: 20

Ingredients:

- 20 mushrooms, stems removed
- 2 cups basil, chopped
- 1 cup tomato sauce, no-salt-added
- 2 tablespoons parsley, chopped
- ¼ cup low-fat parmesan, grated
- 1 and ½ cups whole wheat breadcrumbs
- 1 tablespoon garlic, minced
- ¼ cup low-fat butter, melted
- 2 teaspoons lemon juice
- 1 tablespoon olive oil

Directions:

1. In a bowl, mix butter with breadcrumbs and parsley, stir well and leave aside.
2. In your blender, mix basil with oil, parmesan, garlic and lemon juice and pulse really well.
3. Stuff mushrooms with this mix, pour the tomato sauce on top, sprinkle breadcrumbs mix at the end, cover and cook on Low for 5 hours.
4. Arrange mushrooms on a platter and serve.

Nutrition: Calories 51, Fat 1.1g, Cholesterol 0mg, Sodium 109mg, Carbohydrate 9g, Fiber 1.2g, Sugars 1.1g, Protein 2.2g, Potassium 109mg

Italian Tomato Appetizer

Preparation time: 10 minutes | Cooking time: 2 hours | Servings: 4

Ingredients:

- 2 teaspoons olive oil
- 8 tomatoes, chopped
- 1 garlic clove, minced
- ¼ cup basil, chopped
- 4 Italian whole wheat bread slices, toasted
- 3 tablespoons low-sodium veggie stock
- Black pepper to the taste

Directions:

1. In your slow cooker, mix tomatoes with basil, garlic, oil, stock and black pepper, stir, cover, cook on High for 2 hours and then leave aside to cool down.
2. Divide this mix on the toasted bread and serve as an appetizer.

Nutrition: Calories 158, Fat 4.1g, Cholesterol 0mg, Sodium 251mg, Carbohydrate 26.3g, Fiber 4.5g, Sugars 6.9g, Protein 5.9g, Potassium 590mg

Cauliflower Dip

Preparation time: 10 minutes | Cooking time: 3 hours | Servings: 4

Ingredients:

- ½ pound cauliflower florets
- 1 teaspoon avocado oil
- 1 tablespoon ginger, grated
- 1 cup coconut cream
- 3 garlic cloves, minced
- Black pepper to the taste
- 1 tablespoon basil, chopped
- 1 tablespoon tahini paste
- 1 tablespoon lime juice

Directions:

1. In your slow cooker, combine the cauliflower with the oil, ginger and the other ingredients, put the lid on and cook on Low for 3 hours.
2. Transfer to your blender, pulse well, divide into bowls and serve as a party dip.

Nutrition: Calories 217, Fat 18.1g, Cholesterol 0mg, Sodium 311mg, Carbohydrate 13.3g, Fiber 3.5g, Sugars 5.7g, Protein 3.7g, Potassium 380mg

Sweet Pineapple Snack

Preparation time: 10 minutes | Cooking time: 2 hours | Servings: 8

Ingredients:

- 1 pineapple, peeled and cut into medium sticks
- 2 tablespoons stevia
- 1 tablespoon olive oil
- 1 tablespoon lime juice
- 1 tablespoon lime zest, grated
- 1 teaspoon cinnamon powder
- ¼ teaspoon cloves, ground

Directions:

1. In a bowl, mix lime juice with stevia, oil, cinnamon and cloves and whisk well.
2. Add the pineapple sticks to your slow cooker, add lime mix, toss, cover and cook on High for 2 hours.
3. Serve the pineapple sticks as a snack with lime zest sprinkled on top.

Nutrition: Calories 26, Fat 1.8g, Cholesterol 0mg, Sodium 1mg, Carbohydrate 6.1g, Fiber 0.4g, Sugars 2.1g, Protein 0.1g, Potassium 26mg

Chickpeas Hummus

Preparation time: 10 minutes | Cooking time: 5 hours | Servings: 6

Ingredients:

- 1 cup chickpeas, soaked overnight and drained
- 2 garlic cloves
- ¾ cup green onions, chopped
- 1 tablespoon olive oil
- 2 tablespoons sherry vinegar
- 3 cups water
- 1 teaspoon cumin, ground

Directions:

1. Put the water in your slow cooker, add chickpeas and garlic, cover and cook on Low for 5 hours.
2. Drain chickpeas, transfer them to your blender, add ½ cup of the cooking liquid, green onions, vinegar, oil, cilantro and cumin, blend well, divide into bowls and serve.

Nutrition: Calories 150, Fat 4.5g, Cholesterol 0mg, Sodium 15mg, Carbohydrate 22.3g, Fiber 6.2g, Sugars 3.9g, Protein 6.8g, Potassium 338mg

Asparagus Snack

Preparation time: 4 weeks | Cooking time: 2 hours | Servings: 6

Ingredients:
- 3 cups asparagus spears, halved
- 3 garlic cloves, sliced
- 1 tablespoon dill
- ¼ cup white wine vinegar
- ¼ cup apple cider vinegar
- 2 cloves
- 1 cup water
- ¼ teaspoon red pepper flakes
- 8 black peppercorns
- 1 teaspoon coriander seeds

Directions:
1. In your slow cooker, mix the asparagus with the cider vinegar, white vinegar, dill, cloves, water, garlic, pepper flakes, peppercorns and coriander, cover and cook on High for 2 hours.
2. Drain asparagus, transfer it to bowls and serve as a snack.

Nutrition: Calories 20, Fat 0.1g, Cholesterol 0mg, Sodium 4mg, Carbohydrate 3.6g, Fiber 1.6g, Sugars 1.3g, Protein 1.7g, Potassium 170mg

Shrimp and Beans Appetizer Salad

Preparation time: 10 minutes | Cooking time: 5 hours and 30 minutes | Servings: 8

Ingredients:
- 1 cup tomato, chopped
- ¼ pound shrimp, peeled, deveined and chopped
- 1 cup canned black beans, no-salt-added, drained and rinsed
- 1 cup cucumber, chopped
- 2 teaspoons cumin, ground
- 2 tablespoons olive oil
- ½ cup red onion, chopped
- Zest and juice of 2 limes
- Zest and juice of 2 lemons
- 2 tablespoons garlic, minced
- ¼ cup cilantro, chopped

Directions:

1. In a bowl, mix lime juice and lemon juice with shrimp and toss.
2. Grease the slow cooker with the oil, add black beans, tomato, onion, garlic and cumin, cover and cook on Low for 5 hours.
3. Add shrimp, cover, cook on Low for 30 minutes, more, transfer everything to a bowl, add cucumber and cilantro, toss, leave aside to cool down, divide between small bowls and serve as an appetizer.

Nutrition: Calories 153, Fat 4.4g, Cholesterol 30mg, Sodium 40mg, Carbohydrate 21.4g, Fiber 15.2g, Sugars 2.3g, Protein 9.3g, Potassium 524mg

Mushroom Salsa

Preparation time: 10 minutes | Cooking time: 3 hours | Servings: 4

Ingredients:
- 1 pound white mushrooms, sliced
- 1 cup cherry tomatoes, halved
- 1 cup black olives, pitted and sliced
- 1 tablespoon olive oil
- Juice of 1 lime
- 2 tablespoons parsley, chopped
- 2 tablespoons pumpkin seeds
- 1 tablespoon basil, chopped
- 1 tablespoon balsamic vinegar

Directions:
1. In slow cooker, combine the mushrooms with the tomatoes, olives and the other ingredients, put the lid on and cook on Low for 3 hours.
2. Divide the salsa into bowls and serve as an appetizer.

Nutrition: Calories 129, Fat 9.5g, Cholesterol 0mg, Sodium 304mg, Carbohydrate 9.4g, Fiber 3g, Sugars 3.4g, Protein 5.4g, Potassium 533mg

Pepper and Chickpeas Dip

Preparation time: 10 minutes | Cooking time: 2 hours | Servings: 12

Ingredients:
- 2 cups canned chickpeas, no-salt-added, drained and rinsed
- 1 cup red bell pepper, sliced
- 1 teaspoon onion powder
- 1 tablespoon lemon juice
- 1 teaspoon garlic powder
- 1 tablespoon olive oil
- 2 tablespoons white sesame seeds
- A pinch of cayenne pepper
- 1 and ¼ teaspoons cumin, ground

Directions:
1. In your slow cooker, mix red bell pepper

with oil, sesame seeds, chickpeas, lemon juice, garlic and onion powder, cayenne pepper and cumin, cover and cook on High for 2 hours.
2. Transfer this mix to your blender, pulse well, divide into serving bowls and serve cold.

Nutrition: Calories 143, Fat 3.8g, Cholesterol 0mg, Sodium 9mg, Carbohydrate 21.6g, Fiber 6g, Sugars 4.2g, Protein 6.8g, Potassium 321mg

White Bean Spread

Preparation time: 10 minutes | Cooking time: 6 hours | Servings: 8

Ingredients:
- 15 ounces canned white beans, no-salt-added, drained and rinsed
- 8 garlic cloves, roasted
- 1 cup low-sodium veggie stock
- 2 tablespoons lemon juice
- 2 tablespoons olive oil

Directions:
1. In your blender, mix beans with oil, stock, garlic and lemon juice, cover, cook on Low for 6 hours, transfer to your blender, pulse well, divide into bowls and serve as a snack.

Nutrition: Calories 214, Fat 4g, Cholesterol 0mg, Sodium 19mg, Carbohydrate 33.2g, Fiber 8.2g, Sugars 1.2g, Protein 12.9g, Potassium 971mg

Minty Spinach Dip

Preparation time: 20 minutes | Cooking time: 2 hours | Servings: 4

Ingredients:
- 1 bunch spinach leaves, roughly chopped
- ¾ cup low-fat sour cream
- 1 scallion, sliced
- 2 tablespoons mint leaves, chopped
- Black pepper to the taste

Directions:
1. In your slow cooker, mix the spinach with the scallion, mint, cream and black pepper, cover, cook on High for 2 hours, stir well, divide into bowls and serve.

Nutrition: Calories 121, Fat 9.7g, Cholesterol 19mg, Sodium 147mg, Carbohydrate 6.3g, Fiber 2.2g, Sugars 1g, Protein 4g, Potassium 560mg

Turnips and Cauliflower Spread

Preparation time: 10 minutes | Cooking time: 7 hours | Servings: 4

Ingredients:
- 2 cups cauliflower florets
- 1 cup coconut milk
- 1/3 cup cashews, chopped
- 2 and ½ cups water
- 1 cup turnips, chopped
- 1 teaspoon garlic powder
- ¼ teaspoon smoked paprika
- ¼ teaspoon mustard powder

Directions:
1. In your slow cooker, mix cauliflower with cashews, turnips and water, stir, cover, cook on Low for 7 hours, drain, transfer to a blender, add milk, garlic powder, paprika and mustard powder, blend well, divide into bowls and serve as a snack.

Nutrition: Calories 228, Fat 19.7g, Cholesterol 0mg, Sodium 51mg, Carbohydrate 12.4g, Fiber 3.6g, Sugars 5.2g, Protein 4.6g, Potassium 445mg

Shrimp and Zucchini Salad

Preparation time: 10 minutes | Cooking time: 1 hour | Servings: 4

Ingredients:
- 2 pounds shrimp, peeled and deveined
- ½ cup coconut cream
- 2 tablespoons lime juice
- 1 tablespoon avocado oil
- ½ pound zucchinis, cubed
- 1 cup cherry tomatoes, halved
- 2 tablespoons chives, chopped
- ½ teaspoon oregano, chopped
- 2 garlic cloves, minced

Directions:
1. In the slow cooker, combine the shrimp with the zucchinis, cream and the other ingredients, put the lid on and cook on High for 1 hour.
2. Divide into bowls and serve as an appetizer.

Nutrition: Calories 365, Fat 11.7g, Cholesterol 478mg, Sodium 566mg, Carbohydrate 10.3g, Fiber 2.2g, Sugars 3.4g, Protein 53.7g, Potassium 752mg

Italian Veggie Dip

Preparation time: 10 minutes | Cooking time: 5 hours | Servings: 7

Ingredients:
- 3 cups eggplant, cubed
- 10 ounces white mushrooms, chopped
- 6 garlic cloves, minced
- ½ cauliflower head, riced
- 54 ounces canned tomatoes, no-salt-added and crushed
- 2 tablespoons tomato paste, no-salt-added
- 2 tablespoons stevia
- 2 tablespoons balsamic vinegar
- 1 tablespoon basil, chopped

- 1 and ½ tablespoons oregano, chopped
- A pinch of black pepper

Directions:
1. In your slow cooker, mix cauliflower with tomatoes, mushrooms, eggplant, garlic, stevia, vinegar, tomato paste and pepper, stir, cover and cook on High for 5 hours.
2. Add basil and oregano, stir, mash a bit with a potato masher, divide into bowls and serve as a dip.

Nutrition: Calories 73, Fat 0.8g, Cholesterol 0mg, Sodium 25mg, Carbohydrate 18.9g, Fiber 5.4g, Sugars 8.6g, Protein 4.4g, Potassium 862mg

Cajun Peas Spread

Preparation time: 10 minutes | Cooking time: 5 hours | Servings: 5

Ingredients:
- 3 cups water
- 1 and ½ cups black-eyed peas
- ½ cup pecans, toasted
- ½ teaspoon garlic powder
- ½ teaspoon cayenne powder
- ½ teaspoon chili powder
- 1 teaspoon Cajun seasoning
- A pinch of black pepper

Directions:
1. In your slow cooker, mix the peas with Cajun seasoning, pepper and water, stir, cover and cook on High for 5 hours.
2. Drain, transfer to a blender, add pecans, garlic powder, chili powder and cayenne powder, pulse well, divide into bowls and serve as a snack.

Nutrition: Calories 98, Fat 4.9g, Cholesterol 0mg, Sodium 32mg, Carbohydrate 10.9g, Fiber 3.2g, Sugars 0.3g, Protein 4.3g, Potassium 164mg

Cashew Spread

Preparation time: 10 minutes | Cooking time: 3 hours | Servings: 10

Ingredients:
- 10 ounces hummus, no-salt-added
- 1 cup water
- 1 cup cashews
- 1 teaspoon apple cider vinegar
- ¼ teaspoon garlic powder
- ¼ teaspoon onion powder
- A pinch of black pepper

Directions:
1. In your slow cooker, mix water with cashews and pepper, stir, cover, cook on High for 3 hours, transfer to your blender, add hummus, garlic powder, onion powder and vinegar, pulse well, divide into bowls and serve.

Nutrition: Calories 126, Fat 9.1g, Cholesterol 0mg, Sodium 110mg, Carbohydrate 8.6g, Fiber 2.1g, Sugars 0.7g, Protein 4.4g, Potassium 144mg

Coconut Spinach Dip

Preparation time: 10 minutes | Cooking time: 1 hour | Servings: 4

Ingredients:
- 10 ounces spinach leaves
- 8 ounces water chestnuts, chopped
- 1 cup coconut cream
- 1 garlic clove, minced
- Black pepper to the taste

Directions:
1. In your slow cooker, mix coconut cream with spinach, chestnuts, black pepper and garlic, stir, cover, cook on High for 1 hour, blend with an immersion blender, divide into bowls and serve as a dip

Nutrition: Calories 248, Fat 15.1g, Cholesterol 0mg, Sodium 115mg, Carbohydrate 26.6g, Fiber 2.9g, Sugars 2.7g, Protein 4.8g, Potassium 743mg

Black Bean Salsa

Preparation time: 10 minutes | Cooking time: 4 hours | Servings: 7

Ingredients:
- 1 cup canned black beans, no-salt-added, drained and rinsed
- 1 cup chunky salsa, salt-free
- 6 cups romaine lettuce, torn
- 1 tablespoon low sodium soy sauce
- ½ teaspoon cumin, ground
- ½ cup avocado, peeled, pitted and mashed

Directions:
1. In your slow cooker, mix the beans with salsa, cumin and soy sauce, stir, cover and cook on Low for 4 hours.
2. In a salad bowl, mix lettuce leaves with black beans mix and mashed avocado, toss, divide into small bowls and serve.

Nutrition: Calories 134, Fat 2.6g, Cholesterol 0mg, Sodium 313mg, Carbohydrate 22.2g, Fiber 5.8g, Sugars 2.3g, Protein 7.1g, Potassium 646mg

Mango and Olives Salsa

Preparation time: 10 minutes | Cooking time: 1 hour | Servings: 4

Ingredients:
- 3 mangoes, peeled and roughly cubed
- 1 cup black olives, pitted and halved

- 1 cup kalamata olives, pitted and halved
- 1 cup cherry tomatoes, cubed
- 1 cup corn
- Juice of ½ lemon
- 1 tablespoon olive oil
- 1 teaspoon garlic powder
- 1 tablespoon cilantro, chopped

Directions:
1. In the slow cooker, combine the mango with the olives, tomatoes and the other ingredients, put the lid on and cook on Low for 1 hour.
2. Divide into bowls and serve as an appetizer.

Nutrition: Calories 429, Fat 23.3g, Cholesterol 0mg, Sodium 1258mg, Carbohydrate 57g, Fiber 6.8g, Sugars 37.1g, Protein 4.2g, Potassium 450mg

Chili Coconut Corn Spread

Preparation time: 10 minutes | Cooking time: 2 hours | Servings: 8

Ingredients:
- 8 ounces low-fat cream cheese
- 30 ounces canned corn, no-salt-added, drained
- 2 green onions, chopped
- ½ cup coconut cream
- ½ teaspoon chili powder
- 1 jalapeno, chopped

Directions:
1. In your slow cooker, mix corn with green onions, coconut cream, cream cheese, chili powder and jalapeno, cover, cook on Low for 2 hours, whisk well, divide into bowls and serve as a dip.

Nutrition: Calories 631, Fat 20.3g, Cholesterol 31mg, Sodium 175mg, Carbohydrate 110.8g, Fiber 16.3g, Sugars 19.5g, Protein 21.3g, Potassium 1650mg

Artichoke and Spinach Dip

Preparation time: 10 minutes | Cooking time: 2 hours | Servings: 8

Ingredients:
- 28 ounces canned artichokes, no-salt-added, drained and chopped
- 8 ounces coconut cream
- 10 ounces spinach
- 1 yellow onion, chopped
- ¾ cup coconut milk
- 2 garlic cloves, minced
- 3 tablespoons avocado mayonnaise
- 1 tablespoon red vinegar
- A pinch of black pepper

Directions:
1. In your slow cooker, mix artichokes with spinach, cream, onion, garlic, milk, mayo, vinegar and pepper, stir, cover, cook on Low for 2 hours, divide into bowls and serve as a snack.

Nutrition: Calories 220, Fat 17.6g, Cholesterol 8mg, Sodium 173mg, Carbohydrate 15.6g, Fiber 7.1g, Sugars 2.7g, Protein 5.7g, Potassium 725mg

Mushroom and Bell Pepper Dip

Preparation time: 10 minutes | Cooking time: 4 hours | Servings: 6

Ingredients:
- 1 pound mushrooms, chopped
- 3 cups green bell peppers, chopped
- 28 ounces tomato sauce, no-salt-added
- 1 red onion, chopped
- 3 garlic cloves, minced
- ½ cup low-fat cheddar, grated
- Black pepper to the taste

Directions:
1. In your slow cooker, mix bell peppers with mushrooms, onion, garlic, tomato sauce, cheese and pepper, stir, cover, cook on Low for 4 hours, divide into bowls and serve.

Nutrition: Calories 104, Fat 2g, Cholesterol 0mg, Sodium 737mg, Carbohydrate 17g, Fiber 4g, Sugars 11g, Protein 7.9g, Potassium 823mg

Warm French Veggie Salad

Preparation time: 10 minutes | Cooking time: 9 hours | Servings: 6

Ingredients:
- 6 ounces canned tomato paste, no-salt-added
- 2 tomatoes, cut into medium wedges
- 2 yellow onions, chopped
- 1 eggplant, sliced
- 4 zucchinis, sliced
- 2 green bell peppers, cut into medium strips
- 2 garlic cloves, minced
- 2 tablespoons parsley, chopped
- 3 tablespoons olive oil
- 1 teaspoon oregano, dried
- 1 tablespoon basil, chopped
- A pinch of black pepper

Directions:
1. In your slow cooker, mix oil with onions, eggplant, zucchinis, garlic, bell peppers, tomato paste, tomatoes, basil, oregano and pepper, cover and cook on Low for 9 hours.
2. Add parsley, toss, divide into small bowls and serve warm as an appetizer.

Nutrition: Calories 161, Fat 7.8g, Cholesterol 0mg, Sodium 48mg, Carbohydrate 22.8g, Fiber 7.3g, Sugars 12.7g, Protein 4.9g, Potassium 1047mg

Bulgur and Beans Salad

Preparation time: 10 minutes | Cooking time: 8 hours | Servings: 4

Ingredients:
- 2 cups white mushrooms, sliced
- 14 ounces canned kidney beans, no-salt-added, drained
- 14 ounces canned pinto beans, no-salt-added, drained
- 2 cups yellow onion, chopped
- 1 cup low sodium veggie stock
- 1 cup strong coffee
- ¾ cup bulgur, soaked and drained
- ½ cup red bell pepper, chopped
- 2 garlic cloves, minced
- 2 tablespoons stevia
- 2 tablespoons chili powder
- 1 tablespoon cocoa powder
- 1 teaspoon oregano, dried
- 2 teaspoons cumin, ground
- Black pepper to the taste

Directions:
1. In your slow cooker, mix mushrooms with bulgur, onion, bell pepper, stock, garlic, coffee, kidney and pinto beans, stevia, chili powder, cocoa, oregano, cumin and pepper, stir gently, cover and cook on Low for 12 hours.
2. Divide the mix into small bowls and serve cold as an appetizer.

Nutrition: Calories 837, Fat 4.2g, Cholesterol 0mg, Sodium 165mg, Carbohydrate 162g, Fiber 39.1g, Sugars 9.1g, Protein 49.9g, Potassium 3227mg

Salmon Salad

Preparation time: 10 minutes | Cooking time: 2 hours | Servings: 4

Ingredients:
- 1 pound salmon fillets, boneless and roughly cubed
- Juice of 1 orange
- 1 mango, peeled and cubed
- 1 cup baby spinach
- 1 cup cherry tomatoes, halved
- 1 teaspoon coriander, ground
- 2 tablespoons olive oil
- 2 spring onions, chopped
- 1 red onion, sliced
- 1 Serrano chili pepper, chopped
- ¼ cup cilantro, chopped

Directions:
1. In the slow cooker, combine the salmon with the orange juice, mango and the other ingredients, put the lid on and cook on Low for 2 hours.
2. Divide between appetizer plates and serve.

Nutrition: Calories 300, Fat 14.5g, Cholesterol 50mg, Sodium 61mg, Carbohydrate 20g, Fiber 2.9g, Sugars 15.8g, Protein 23.9g, Potassium 829mg

Pineapple Chicken Wings

Preparation time: 10 minutes | Cooking time: 3 hours | Servings: 6

Ingredients:
- 3 pounds chicken wings
- 2 and ¼ cups pineapple juice, unsweetened
- 1 teaspoon olive oil
- 3 tablespoons low sodium soy sauce
- 2 tablespoons almond flour
- 2 tablespoons garlic, minced
- 1 tablespoon ginger, minced
- 2 tablespoons 5 spice powder
- A pinch of red pepper flakes, crushed

Directions:
1. Put the pineapple juice in your slow cooker, add the oil, ginger, soy sauce, garlic and flour and whisk really well.
2. Season chicken wings with pepper flakes and 5-spice powder, add them to your slow cooker, cover and cook on High for 3 hours.
3. Transfer chicken wings to a platter, drizzle some of the sauce over them and serve as an appetizer.

Nutrition: Calories 568, Fat 23.2g, Cholesterol 202mg, Sodium 506mg, Carbohydrate 18.4g, Fiber 1.4g, Sugars 11.7g, Protein 68.7g, Potassium 713mg

Spiced Pecans Snack

Preparation time: 10 minutes | Cooking time: 2 hours | Servings: 5

Ingredients:
- 1 pound pecans, halved
- 1 tablespoon chili powder
- 2 tablespoons olive oil
- 1 teaspoon basil, dried
- 1 teaspoon oregano, dried
- ½ teaspoon onion powder
- ¼ teaspoon garlic powder
- 1 teaspoon rosemary, dried

Directions:
1. In your slow cooker, mix pecans with oil, basil, chili powder, oregano, garlic powder, onion powder and rosemary, toss, cover and cook on Low for 2 hours.
2. Divide into bowls and serve as a snack.

Nutrition: Calories 688, Fat 70.7g, Cholesterol 0mg, Sodium 16mg, Carbohydrate 14.4g, Fiber 10.5g, Sugars 3.5g, Protein 10g, Potassium 416mg

Beef Party Meatballs

Preparation time: 10 minutes | Cooking time: 4 hours | Servings: 4

Ingredients:
- 14 ounces coconut milk
- 1 egg, whisked
- 1 and ½ pounds beef, minced
- 2 small yellow onions, chopped
- 3 tablespoons cilantro, chopped
- 2 tablespoons chili powder
- 1 teaspoon basil, dried
- 1 tablespoon green curry paste
- 1 tablespoon low sodium soy sauce
- Black pepper to the taste

Directions:
1. Put the meat in a bowl, add onion, egg, pepper and cilantro, stir well, shape medium-sized meatballs and place them in your slow cooker.
2. Add chili powder, soy sauce, milk, curry paste and basil, toss and cook on Low for 4 hours.
3. Arrange meatballs on a platter and serve them as an appetizer.

Nutrition: Calories 606, Fat 37.1g, Cholesterol 193mg, Sodium 538mg, Carbohydrate 13.3g, Fiber 4.3g, Sugars 5.7g, Protein 56.4g, Potassium 1096mg

Beef Rolls

Preparation time: 10 minutes | Cooking time: 8 hours | Servings: 4

Ingredients:
- 25 ounces tomato sauce, no-salt-added
- 1 cup cauliflower rice
- 1 green cabbage head, leaves separated
- ½ cup onion, chopped
- 2 ounces white mushrooms, chopped
- ½ pounds beef meat, minced
- 2 garlic cloves, minced
- ¼ cup water
- 2 tablespoons dill, chopped
- 1 tablespoon olive oil
- A pinch of black pepper

Directions:
1. In a bowl, mix beef with onion, cauliflower, mushrooms, garlic, dill and pepper and stir.
2. Arrange cabbage leaves on a working surface, divide the beef mix and wrap them well.
3. Add sauce and water to your slow cooker, stir, add cabbage rolls, cover, cook on Low for 8 hours, arrange the rolls on a platter and serve them as an appetizer.

Nutrition: Calories 243, Fat 8.3g, Cholesterol 43mg, Sodium 1033mg, Carbohydrate 24.8g, Fiber 7.8g, Sugars 15.1g, Protein 21.5g, Potassium 1211mg

Shrimp Dip

Preparation time: 10 minutes | Cooking time: 1 hour | Servings: 4

Ingredients:
- 1 pound shrimp, peeled, deveined, cooked and chopped
- 1 cup low-fat cream cheese
- 1 cup coconut cream
- ½ cup low-fat cheddar, shredded
- 3 spring onions, chopped
- 1 tablespoon mustard
- 1 tablespoon lime juice
- 1 teaspoon turmeric powder

Directions:
1. In the slow cooker, combine the shrimp with the cream cheese and the other ingredients, put the lid on and cook on High for 1 hour.
2. Divide into small bowls and serve as a party dip.

Nutrition: Calories 373, Fat 18.9g, Cholesterol 246mg, Sodium 691mg, Carbohydrate 11.4g, Fiber 2.2g, Sugars 2.9g, Protein 40g, Potassium 525mg

Tomato Salsa

Preparation time: 10 minutes | Cooking time: 7 hours | Servings: 4

Ingredients:
- 8 ounces black olives, pitted and sliced
- 3 cups tomatoes, chopped
- 1 red onion, chopped
- 2 tablespoons mint, chopped
- 2 teaspoons capers, no-salt-added
- 2 teaspoons balsamic vinegar
- Black pepper to the taste

Directions:
1. In your slow cooker, mix tomatoes with capers, olives, onion, vinegar, mint and pepper, toss, cover and cook on Low for 7 hours.
2. Divide salsa into small bowls and serve cold.

Nutrition: Calories 109, Fat 6.7g, Cholesterol 0mg, Sodium 601mg, Carbohydrate 12.6g, Fiber 4.3g, Sugars 5.2g, Protein 2.1g, Potassium 380mg

White Fish Sticks

Preparation time: 10 minutes | Cooking time: 2 hours | Servings: 4

Ingredients:

- 2 eggs
- 1 pound white fish fillets, skinless, boneless and cut into medium strips
- Black pepper to the taste
- 1 cup almond flour
- ¼ teaspoon paprika
- Cooking spray

Directions:

1. In a bowl, mix the flour with pepper and paprika and stir.
2. Put the eggs in another bowl and whisk them well
3. Dip fish sticks in the egg, dredge in flour mix, arrange them in your slow cooker greased with cooking spray, cover and cook on High for 2 hours.
4. Serve them as an appetizer.

Nutrition: Calories 403, Fat 24.5g, Cholesterol 169mg, Sodium 171mg, Carbohydrate 7.1g, Fiber 3.1g, Sugars 0.6g, Protein 36.6g, Potassium 493mg

Tomato Shrimp Salad

Preparation time: 10 minutes | Cooking time: 3 hours | Servings: 4

Ingredients:

- 3 pounds shrimp, peeled and deveined
- 14 ounces canned tomato paste, no-salt-added
- 1 red onion, chopped

Directions:

1. In your slow cooker, mix shrimp with onion and tomato paste, stir, cover and cook on Low for 3 hours.
2. Divide into small bowls and serve.

Nutrition: Calories 497, Fat 6.3g, Cholesterol 716mg, Sodium 928mg, Carbohydrate 26.5g, Fiber 4.7g, Sugars 13.3g, Protein 82.1g, Potassium 1623mg

Green Beans Salsa

Preparation time: 10 minutes | Cooking time: 2 hours | Servings: 4

Ingredients:

- 1 pound green beans, trimmed and halved
- 1 cup corn
- 1 cup black olives, pitted and halved
- 2 tablespoons balsamic vinegar
- 1 cup cherry tomatoes, halved
- 2 tablespoons olive oil
- 2 garlic cloves, minced
- 1 teaspoon rosemary, dried
- ½ cup low-sodium veggie stock

Directions:

1. In your slow cooker, combine the green beans with the corn, olives and the other ingredients, put the lid on and cook on High for 2 hours.
2. Divide into bowls and serve as an appetizer.

Nutrition: Calories 182, Fat 11.3g, Cholesterol 0mg, Sodium 357mg, Carbohydrate 20.5g, Fiber 6.7g, Sugars 4.2g, Protein 4.1g, Potassium 465mg

Stuffed Chicken

Preparation time: 10 minutes | Cooking time: 6 hours | Servings: 4

Ingredients:

- 4 chicken breasts, skinless and boneless
- 1 tablespoon olive oil
- 1 small yellow onion, chopped
- 2 chili peppers, chopped
- 1 red bell pepper, chopped
- 2 teaspoons garlic, minced
- 6 ounces spinach
- 1 tablespoon lemon juice
- 1 cup low-sodium veggie stock
- A pinch of black pepper
- A handful parsley, chopped

Directions:

1. Heat up a pan with the oil over medium-high heat, add bell pepper, chili peppers, onions, spinach, garlic, pepper and oregano, stir, cook for a couple of minutes and take off heat
2. Cut a pocket in each chicken breast, stuff with spinach mix, arrange in your slow cooker, add the stock, cover, cook on Low for 6 hours, arrange stuffed chicken on a platter, sprinkle parsley on top, drizzle the lemon juice and serve as an appetizer.

Nutrition: Calories 342, Fat 14.7g, Cholesterol 130mg, Sodium 181mg, Carbohydrate 6.6g, Fiber 2g, Sugars 2.6g, Protein 44.7g, Potassium 702mg

Italian Nuts Mix

Preparation time: 10 minutes | Cooking time: 4 hours | Servings: 20

Ingredients:

- 4 tablespoons olive oil
- 1-ounce Italian seasoning
- Cayenne pepper to the taste
- 2 cups almonds
- 2 cups walnuts
- 2 cups cashews
- 1 teaspoon cinnamon powder

Directions:

1. In your slow cooker, mix oil with Italian seasoning, cinnamon, cayenne, cashews, almonds and walnuts, toss well, cover, cook on Low for 4 hours, divide into bowls and serve as a snack.

Nutrition: Calories 240, Fat 21.7g, Cholesterol 1mg, Sodium 3mg, Carbohydrate 8.1g, Fiber 2.5g, Sugars 1.4g, Protein 7.2g, Potassium 213mg

Dill Walnuts and Seeds Mix

Preparation time: 10 minutes | Cooking time: 3 hours | Servings: 10

Ingredients:

- 1 cup walnuts, chopped
- 1 cup pumpkin seeds
- Cooking spray
- 2 tablespoons olive oil
- 2 tablespoons dill, dried
- 1 tablespoon lemon peel, grated
- 1 teaspoon rosemary, dried

Directions:

1. Spray your slow cooker with cooking spray, add walnuts, pumpkin seeds, oil, dill, rosemary and lemon peel, toss, cover, cook on Low for 3 hours, divide into bowls and serve as a snack.

Nutrition: Calories 179, Fat 16.6g, Cholesterol 0mg, Sodium 4mg, Carbohydrate 4.3g, Fiber 1.6g, Sugars 0.3g, Protein 6.5g, Potassium 200mg

Kale Dip

Preparation time: 10 minutes | Cooking time: 1 hour | Servings: 4

Ingredients:

- 1 pound baby kale
- 1 cup coconut cream
- 2 spring onions, chopped
- 1 cup low-fat cream cheese
- 1 scallion, chopped
- 2 tablespoons mint leaves, chopped
- A pinch of cayenne pepper
- A pinch of red pepper flakes, crushed

Directions:

1. In your slow cooker, combine the kale with the cream, spring onions and the other ingredients, put the lid on and cook on Low for 1 hour.
2. Blend using an immersion blender, divide into bowls and serve as a party dip.

Nutrition: Calories 404, Fat 35.2g, Cholesterol 64mg, Sodium 229mg, Carbohydrate 17.4g, Fiber 4.4g, Sugars 2.3g, Protein 10g, Potassium 262mg

Tomato Dip

Preparation time: 10 minutes | Cooking time: 5 hours | Servings: 12

Ingredients:

- 8 pounds tomatoes, peeled and chopped
- 6 ounces tomato paste, no-salt-added
- ¼ cup white vinegar
- 2 sweet onions, chopped
- 1 and ½ tablespoons Italian seasoning
- 2 tablespoons stevia
- ½ cup basil, chopped
- A pinch of black pepper

Directions:

1. In your slow cooker, mix the tomatoes with onions, tomato paste, vinegar, stevia, Italian seasoning, pepper and basil, stir, cover, cook on High for 5 hours, blend using an immersion blender, divide into bowls and serve as a dip.

Nutrition: Calories 80, Fat 1.2g, Cholesterol 1mg, Sodium 30mg, Carbohydrate 18.5g, Fiber 4.6g, Sugars 10.6g, Protein 3.5g, Potassium 895mg

Zucchini Dip

Preparation time: 10 minutes | Cooking time: 2 hours | Servings: 4

Ingredients:

- 4 cups zucchinis, chopped
- 1 cup low-sodium chicken stock
- 4 garlic cloves, minced
- ¾ cup sesame paste
- ¼ cup olive oil
- ½ cup lemon juice
- Black pepper to the taste

Directions:

1. In your slow cooker, mix the zucchinis with stock and pepper, cover, cook on High for 2 hours, transfer to your blender, add oil, garlic, lemon juice and sesame paste, blend, divide into small bowls and serve.

Nutrition: Calories 425, Fat 37.7g, Cholesterol 0mg, Sodium 99mg, Carbohydrate 17.6g, Fiber 4.1g, Sugars 3g, Protein 10.8g, Potassium 625mg

Easy Zucchini Rolls

Preparation time: 10 minutes | Cooking time: 1 hour | Servings: 24

Ingredients:

- 2 tablespoons olive oil
- 24 basil leaves
- 3 zucchinis, thinly sliced
- ½ cup tomato sauce, no-salt-added
- ¼ cup basil leaves, whole
- 2 tablespoons mint, chopped
- 1 and ½ cup low-fat ricotta cheese
- Black pepper to the taste

Directions:

1. Brush zucchini slices with half of the olive oil, season with the pepper and place them on a working surface.
2. In a bowl, mix ricotta with chopped basil,

mint and pepper, stir well, spread this over zucchini, divide whole basil leaves, roll them, transfer to your slow cooker add the rest of the oil and the tomato sauce, cover, cook on High for 1 hour, arrange them on a platter and serve.

Nutrition: Calories 41, Fat 2.6g, Cholesterol 5mg, Sodium 56mg, Carbohydrate 2.9g, Fiber 1g, Sugars 0.8g, Protein 2.4g, Potassium 152mg

Jumbo Shrimp Appetizer

Preparation time: 10 minutes | Cooking time: 1 hour | Servings: 4

Ingredients:

1 pound jumbo shrimp, peeled and deveined

1 and ½ cups low-sodium chicken stock

Juice of 1 lemon

2 teaspoons Creole seasoning

4 teaspoons cider vinegar

4 teaspoons avocado oil

Black pepper to the taste

Directions:

1. Grease your slow cooker with the oil, add shrimp, vinegar, stock, lemon juice, pepper and Creole seasoning, cover, cook on High for 1 hour, transfer the shrimp to a platter and serve as an appetizer.

Nutrition: Calories 98, Fat 0.9g, Cholesterol 233mg, Sodium 1952mg, Carbohydrate 1.2g, Fiber 0.3g, Sugars 2.7g, Protein 20.8g, Potassium 33mg

Black Beans Salsa

Preparation time: 10 minutes | Cooking time: 4 hours | Servings: 4

Ingredients:

- 2 cups canned black beans, no-salt added, drained and rinsed
- 1 cup corn
- 1 cup kalamata olives, pitted and halved
- 1 cup baby spinach
- 1 cup cherry tomatoes, halved
- 1 cup spring onions, chopped
- 1 cup low-sodium veggie stock
- 1 tablespoon balsamic vinegar
- 1 tablespoon avocado oil
- 2 tablespoons lemon juice

Directions:

1. In the slow cooker, combine the black beans with the corn, olives and the other ingredients except the spinach, put the lid on and cook on Low for 3 hours and 30 minutes.
2. Add the spinach, cook the mix for 30 minutes more on Low, divide into bowls and serve as an appetizer.

Nutrition: Calories 431, Fat 6.1g, Cholesterol 0mg, Sodium 353mg, Carbohydrate 76.4g, Fiber 18.4g, Sugars 5.5g, Protein 23.7g, Potassium 1786mg

Salmon Appetizer Salad

Preparation time: 10 minutes | Cooking time: 1 hour | Servings: 4

Ingredients:

- 4 medium salmon fillets, boneless and cubed
- 2 shallots, chopped
- 1 cup low sodium veggie stock
- 1 lettuce head, torn
- ¼ cup olive oil+ 1 tablespoon
- 2 tablespoons lemon juice
- 3 tablespoons parsley, finely chopped
- Black pepper to the taste

Directions:

1. Brush salmon fillets with 1 tablespoon of oil, season with pepper, put them in your slow cooker, add stock, cover and cook on High for 1 hour.
2. Transfer salmon to a salad bowl, add shallots, lemon juice, lettuce, the rest of the oil and parsley, toss and serve as an appetizer.

Nutrition: Calories 407, Fat 28.3g, Cholesterol 78mg, Sodium 178mg, Carbohydrate 5g, Fiber 0.7g, Sugars 1.7g, Protein 35.2g, Potassium 840mg

Beet and Celery Spread

Preparation time: 10 minutes | Cooking time: 4 hours | Servings: 8

Ingredients:

- 6 beets, peeled and chopped
- 1 yellow onion, chopped
- 1 cup low-sodium veggie stock
- ¼ cup lemon juice
- 2 tablespoons olive oil
- 7 celery ribs
- 8 garlic cloves, minced
- 1 bunch basil, chopped
- Black pepper to the taste

Directions:

1. Grease your slow cooker with the oil, add celery, onion, beets, garlic, stock, lemon juice, basil and pepper, stir, cover and cook on Low for 4 hours.
2. Blend using an immersion blender, divide into bowls and serve.

Nutrition: Calories 171, Fat 7.9g, Cholesterol 0mg, Sodium 250mg, Carbohydrate 23g, Fiber 5g, Sugars 14.9g, Protein 4.4g, Potassium 727mg

Clams Salad

Preparation time: 10 minutes | Cooking time: 2 hours | Servings: 4

Ingredients:
- 10 ounces low sodium veggie stock
- 40 small clams
- Lemon wedges for serving
- 1 yellow onion, chopped
- 2 tablespoons parsley, chopped
- 1 teaspoon olive oil

Directions:
1. Grease your slow cooker with the oil; add onion, clams, stock and parsley, toss, cover and cook on High for 2 hours.
2. Divide into small bowls and serve with lemon wedges on the side.

Nutrition: Calories 172, Fat 1.8g, Cholesterol 0mg, Sodium 1137mg, Carbohydrate 36.5g, Fiber 1.9g, Sugars 11.5g, Protein 2.2g, Potassium 322mg

Creamy Endive Salad

Preparation time: 10 minutes | Cooking time: 3 hours | Servings: 4

Ingredients:
- 1 cup low-sodium chicken stock
- 4 endives, trimmed
- 14 ounces coconut cream
- 4 slices low-sodium ham, chopped
- 2 tablespoons olive oil
- ½ teaspoon nutmeg, ground
- Black pepper to the taste

Directions:
1. In your slow cooker, mix endives with stock, pepper, oil, ham, nutmeg and coconut cream, cover and cook on High for 3 hours.
2. Divide into small bowls and serve as an appetizer.

Nutrition: Calories 347, Fat 33.5g, Cholesterol 16mg, Sodium 475mg, Carbohydrate 8.4g, Fiber 3.4g, Sugars .3.9g, Protein 7.6g, Potassium 421mg

Chili Cauliflower Dip

Preparation time: 10 minutes | Cooking time: 2 hours and 15 minutes | Servings: 6

Ingredients:
- 2 cups cauliflower rice
- 2 jalapenos, chopped
- ½ cup coconut cream
- 2 tablespoons chives, chopped
- ¼ cup low-fat cheddar cheese, grated
- A pinch of black pepper

Directions:
1. In your slow cooker, mix the jalapenos with the coconut cream, cauliflower, pepper, cheese and chives, stir, cover and cook on Low for 2 hours and 15 minutes.
2. Divide into bowls and serve.

Nutrition: Calories 85, Fat 7g, Cholesterol 5mg, Sodium 72mg, Carbohydrate 3.7g, Fiber 0.6g, Sugars .2.2g, Protein 3g, Potassium 70mg

Cranberries, Apple and Onion Salad

Preparation time: 10 minutes | Cooking time: 6 hours | Servings: 12

Ingredients:
- 2 cups sweet onions, sliced
- 1 apple, peeled, cored and cut into wedges
- ½ cup cranberries
- ¼ cup balsamic vinegar
- 2 tablespoons olive oil
- 1 tablespoon stevia
- ½ teaspoon orange zest, grated
- 7 ounces low-fat cheddar cheese, shredded

Directions:
1. In your slow cooker, mix apples with cranberries, onions, oil, vinegar, stevia and orange zest, stir, cover and cook on Low for 6 hours.
2. Divide into bowls, sprinkle the cheese on top and serve.

Nutrition: Calories 108, Fat 7.9g, Cholesterol 17mg, Sodium 104mg, Carbohydrate 5.7g, Fiber 1g, Sugars .3g, Protein 4.4g, Potassium 76mg

Sausage Meatballs and Apricot Sauce

Preparation time: 10 minutes | Cooking time: 5 hours | Servings: 20

Ingredients:
- 12 ounces canned apricot preserves, unsweetened
- 2 pounds beef sausage, ground
- 2 eggs
- ½ cup yellow onion, chopped
- 2 tablespoons parsley, chopped
- ½ teaspoon garlic powder
- A pinch of black pepper

Directions:
1. In a bowl, mix beef sausage meat with eggs, onion, parsley, pepper and garlic powder, stir well and shape small meatballs out of this mix.
2. Put the meatballs in your slow cooker, add apricot preserves, toss, cover and cook on Low for 5 hours.
3. Arrange meatballs, sauce on a platter, and serve them.

Nutrition: Calories 229, Fat 16.9g, Cholesterol 49mg, Sodium 378mg, Carbohydrate 12.6g, Fiber 0.1g, Sugars 7.6g, Protein 7g, Potassium 112mg

Sriracha Chicken Dip

Preparation time: 10 minutes | Cooking time: 3 hours and 30 minutes | Servings: 10

Ingredients:

- 8 ounces coconut cream
- 1 pound chicken breast, skinless, boneless and sliced
- ¼ cup low-sodium chicken stock
- 3 tablespoons jalapeno pepper powder
- 2 tablespoons stevia
- 1 teaspoon chili powder

Directions:

1. In your slow cooker, mix chicken with jalapeno pepper, stock, stevia and chili powder, stir, cover and cook on High for 3 hours.
2. Shred meat, return to pot, add coconut cream, cover, cook on High for 30 minutes more, divide into bowls and serve.

Nutrition: Calories 105, Fat 6.6g, Cholesterol 29mg, Sodium 33mg, Carbohydrate 3.5g, Fiber 0.6g, Sugars 0.8g, Protein 10.2g, Potassium 232mg

Shrimp Cocktail

Preparation time: 10 minutes | Cooking time: 2 hours and 30 minutes | Servings: 4

Ingredients:

- 1 cup low-sodium chicken stock
- 40 shrimp, peeled and deveined
- 2 tablespoons olive oil
- 2 teaspoons garlic, minced
- 2 teaspoons parsley, chopped

Directions:

1. In your slow cooker, mix stock with oil, parsley, garlic and shrimp, toss, cover and cook on Low for 2 hours and 30 minutes.
2. Divide into bowls and serve as an appetizer.

Nutrition: Calories 325, Fat 10.7g, Cholesterol 463mg, Sodium 571mg, Carbohydrate 3.8g, Fiber 0.1g, Sugars 0g, Protein 50.5g, Potassium 382mg

Cod Salsa

Preparation time: 10 minutes | Cooking time: 1 hour and 30 minutes | Servings: 4

Ingredients:

- 15 ounces canned tomatoes, no-salt-added and chopped
- 1 pound cod fillets, skinless, boneless and cubed
- 1 red bell pepper, chopped
- 1 yellow onion, chopped
- 1 tablespoons rosemary, chopped
- ¼ cup low sodium veggie stock

Directions:

1. In your slow cooker, mix tomatoes with onion, bell pepper, rosemary and stock and stir.
2. Add fish, cover and cook on Low for 1 hour and 30 minutes.
3. Divide everything into bowls and serve warm as an appetizer.

Nutrition: Calories 134, Fat 1.5g, Cholesterol 56mg, Sodium 103mg, Carbohydrate 9.7g, Fiber 2.6g, Sugars 5.5g, Protein 21.8g, Potassium 356mg

Salmon and Carrots Appetizer Salad

Preparation time: 10 minutes | Cooking time: 9 hours | Servings: 4

Ingredients:

- 16 ounces baby carrots
- 4 salmon fillets, boneless and cubed
- 3 tablespoons olive oil
- ¼ cup low-sodium veggie stock
- ½ teaspoon dill, chopped
- 4 garlic cloves, minced
- A pinch of black pepper

Directions:

1. In your slow cooker, mix oil with carrots, stock and garlic, stir, cover and cook on Low for 7 hours.
2. Add salmon, pepper and dill, cover, cook on Low for 2 hours more, divide everything into bowls and serve as an appetizer

Nutrition: Calories 371, Fat 21.7g, Cholesterol 78mg, Sodium 176mg, Carbohydrate 10.5g, Fiber 3.4g, Sugars 5.5g, Protein 35.5g, Potassium 969mg

Italian Shrimp Salad

Preparation time: 10 minutes | Cooking time: 8 hours | Servings: 8

Ingredients:

- 4 cups low-sodium veggie stock
- 1 pound sausage, no extra salt added and sliced
- 2 pounds shrimp, deveined
- 2 tablespoons Italian seasoning
- 2 tablespoons parsley, chopped
- 4 tablespoons olive oil
- A pinch of black pepper

Directions:

1. In your slow cooker, mix stock with Italian

seasoning, sausage, pepper, oil and shrimp, toss, cover, cook on Low for 8 hours, add parsley, toss, divide into small bowls and serve as an appetizer.

Nutrition: Calories 406, Fat 26.1g, Cholesterol 289mg, Sodium 773mg, Carbohydrate 3.2g, Fiber 0g, Sugars 0.8g, Protein 36.9g, Potassium 366mg

Salmon and Scallions Salad

Preparation time: 10 minutes | Cooking time: 2 hours | Servings: 4

Ingredients:
- 3 salmon fillets, skin on, boneless and cubed
- Zest of 1 lemon, grated
- 2 cups low-sodium chicken stock
- ¼ cup dill, chopped
- 4 scallions, chopped
- 3 black peppercorns
- ½ teaspoon fennel seeds
- 1 teaspoon white wine vinegar
- Black pepper to the taste

Directions:
1. In your slow cooker, mix lemon zest with scallions, peppercorns, fennel, pepper, vinegar, stock, dill and salmon, cover and cook on High for 2 hours.
2. Divide salmon and scallions salad into bowls and serve warm as an appetizer.

Nutrition: Calories 200, Fat 8.7g, Cholesterol 59mg, Sodium 191mg, Carbohydrate 4.1g, Fiber 1.1g, Sugars 0.9g, Protein 27.4g, Potassium 662mg

Salmon Bites and Lemon Dressing

Preparation time: 10 minutes | Cooking time: 2 hours | Servings: 4

Ingredients:
- 4 salmon fillets, skinless, boneless and cubed
- 1 lemon, sliced
- 1 cup low-sodium veggie stock
- 2 tablespoons chili pepper
- Juice of 1 lemon
- 1 teaspoon basil, dried
- 1 teaspoon sweet paprika
- Salt and black pepper to the taste

Directions:
1. In your slow cooker, mix chili pepper with lemon juice, stock, paprika, basil, pepper and salmon, cover and cook on High for 2 hours.
2. Divide salmon into bowls drizzle sauce from the pot all over and serve.

Nutrition: Calories 284, Fat 12.8g, Cholesterol 78mg, Sodium 380mg, Carbohydrate 7g, Fiber 1.1g, Sugars 3.4g, Protein 35.7g, Potassium 753mg

Dash Diet Slow Cooker Dessert Recipes

Easy Carrot and Pineapple Cake

Preparation time: 10 minutes | Cooking time: 2 hours and 30 minutes | Servings: 6

Ingredients:
- 1 cup pineapple, dried and chopped
- 4 carrots, chopped
- 1 cup dates, pitted and chopped
- ½ cup coconut flakes
- Cooking spray
- 1 and ½ cups whole wheat flour
- ½ teaspoon cinnamon powder

Directions:
1. Put carrots in your food processor and pulse.
2. Add flour, dates, pineapple, coconut, cinnamon, and pulse very well again.
3. Grease the slow cooker with the cooking spray, pour the cake mix, spread, cover and cook on High for 2 hours and 30 minutes.
4. Leave the cake to cool down, slice and serve.

Nutrition: Calories 252, Fat 2.8g, Cholesterol 0mg, Sodium 31mg, Carbohydrate 54.7g, Fiber 5.2g, Sugars 24g, Protein 4.7g, Potassium 412mg

Mango Cake

Preparation time: 10 minutes | Cooking time: 2 hours and 30 minutes | Servings: 6

Ingredients:
- 1 cup mango, peeled and chopped
- 1 and ½ cups whole wheat flour
- ½ cup coconut milk
- 1 cup avocado, peeled, pitted and mashed
- ½ cup coconut flakes, unsweetened
- ½ teaspoon cinnamon powder

Directions:
1. In a bowl mix the mango with the flour and the other ingredients and whisk.
2. Line the slow cooker with parchment paper, pour the cake mix and cook on High fro 2 hours and 30 minutes.
3. Cool the cake down before slicing and serving it.

Nutrition: Calories 249, Fat 12.2g, Cholesterol 0mg, Sodium 7mg, Carbohydrate 32.2g, Fiber 4g, Sugars 5g, Protein 4.6g, Potassium 274mg

Coconut Green Tea Cream

Preparation time: 10 minutes | Cooking time: 1 hour | Servings: 4

Ingredients:
- 1 cup fat-free coconut cream
- 4 tablespoons low-fat coconut milk
- 4 and ½ teaspoons green tea powder
- 3 tablespoons hot water

Directions:
1. In a bowl, mix green tea powder with hot water, stir well and leave aside to cool down.
2. In your slow cooker, mix the green tea with milk and cream, stir, cover, cook on High for 1 hour, transfer to a container and freeze before serving.

Nutrition: Calories 80, Fat 4.2g, Cholesterol 0mg, Sodium 21mg, Carbohydrate 8.1g, Fiber 1g, Sugars 6.3g, Protein 1.9g, Potassium 87mg

Sweet Coconut Figs

Preparation time: 6 minutes | Cooking time: 2 hours | Servings: 4

Ingredients:
- 1 cup coconut cream
- 12 figs, halved
- 2 tablespoons coconut butter, melted
- ¼ cup palm sugar

Directions:
1. In your slow cooker, mix the coconut butter with the figs, sugar and cream, stir, cover and cook on High for 2 hours.
2. Divide into bowls and serve cold.

Nutrition: Calories 353, Fat 19.3g, Cholesterol 0mg, Sodium 322mg, Carbohydrate 47.7g, Fiber 8.2g, Sugars 35.7g, Protein 3.8g, Potassium 802mg

Avocado and Cashews Cake

Preparation time: 10 minutes | Cooking time: 2 hours and 30 minutes | Servings: 6

Ingredients:
- 1 and ½ cups avocado, peeled, pitted and mashed
- ½ cup coconut milk
- ½ cup coconut cream
- ½ teaspoon vanilla extract
- 1 cup cashews, chopped
- 4 tablespoons avocado oil
- Juice of 2 limes
- 2 tablespoons coconut sugar

Directions:
1. In your food processor, combine the avocado with the cream and the other ingredients and pulse well.
2. Pour this into the slow cooker lined with parchment paper and cook on High for 2 hours and 30 minutes.
3. Slice and serve cold.

Nutrition: Calories 250, Fat 19.1g, Cholesterol 0mg, Sodium 16mg, Carbohydrate 22.4g, Fiber 4.4g, Sugars 14.4g, Protein 2g, Potassium 390mg

Chocolate and Vanilla Cream

Preparation time: 1 hour and 10 minutes | Cooking time: 2 hours | Servings: 4

Ingredients:
- 2 cups low-fat milk
- 3 ounces dark and unsweetened chocolate
- 1 cup warm water
- 3 tablespoons stevia
- 2 tablespoons gelatin
- 1 tablespoon vanilla extract

Directions:
1. In a bowl, mix warm water with gelatin, stir well and leave aside for 1 hour.
2. Put this in your slow cooker, add milk, stevia, chocolate and vanilla, stir well, cover, cook on High for 2 hours, whisk the cream one more time, divide into bowls and serve.

Nutrition: Calories 181, Fat 12.8g, Cholesterol 6mg, Sodium 65mg, Carbohydrate 19.4g, Fiber 3.5g, Sugars 6.8g, Protein 10.4g, Potassium 189mg

Cinnamon Tomato Mix

Preparation time: 10 minutes | Cooking time: 4 hours | Servings: 4

Ingredients:
- 5 pounds tomatoes, blanched and peeled
- 3 cups water, hot
- 3 cups coconut sugar
- 2 cinnamon sticks
- ½ teaspoon cinnamon powder
- 2 teaspoons vanilla extract
- ½ teaspoon cloves, ground

Directions:
1. In your slow cooker, mix the tomatoes with the water, cinnamon sticks, cinnamon powder, sugar, vanilla and cloves, stir, cover and cook on Low for 4 hours.
2. Discard cinnamon sticks, leave the tomatoes aside to cool down, divide into bowls and serve!

Nutrition: Calories 183, Fat 1.2g, Cholesterol 0mg, Sodium 64mg, Carbohydrate 37.7g, Fiber 7.5g, Sugars 15.2g, Protein 5.8g, Potassium 1356mg

Tomato Pie

Preparation time: 10 minutes | Cooking time: 3 hours | Servings: 6

Ingredients:
- 1 cup tomatoes, blanched, peeled and chopped
- ½ cup olive oil
- 1 and ½ cups whole

- wheat flour
- Cooking spray
- 1 teaspoon cinnamon powder
- 1 teaspoon baking soda
- 1 teaspoon baking powder
- ¾ cup coconut sugar
- 2 tablespoons apple cider vinegar

Directions:
1. In a bowl, mix flour with sugar, cinnamon, baking powder and soda and stir well.
2. In another bowl, mix tomatoes with oil and cider vinegar and stir very well.
3. Combine the 2 mixtures, stir, pour everything into your slow cooker greased with cooking spray, cover and cook on High for 3 hours.
4. Leave the pie aside to cool down, slice and serve.

Nutrition: Calories 412, Fat 25.9g, Cholesterol 0mg, Sodium 327mg, Carbohydrate 41.7g, Fiber 1.8g, Sugars 1.3g, Protein 5.4g, Potassium 289mg

Mint Cream

Preparation time: 10 minutes | Cooking time: 1 hour | Servings: 4

Ingredients:
- 1 cup almond milk
- 1 tablespoon coconut sugar
- 1 teaspoon maple syrup
- 1 tablespoon mint, chopped
- 1 cup fat-free coconut cream
- 2 teaspoons green tea powder

Directions:
1. In the slow cooker, combine the milk with the sugar and the other ingredients, put the lid on and cook on High for 1 hour.
2. Divide into bowls and serve cold.

Nutrition: Calories 241, Fat 16.1g, Cholesterol 5mg, Sodium 134mg, Carbohydrate 21.8g, Fiber 2.1g, Sugars 3g, Protein 4.3g, Potassium 293mg

Berries and Orange Sauce

Preparation time: 10 minutes | Cooking time: 2 hours | Servings: 4

Ingredients:
- 1 cup orange juice
- 1 pound strawberries, halved
- 2 cups blueberries
- 1 and ½ tablespoons stevia
- 1 tablespoon olive oil
- 1 and ½ tablespoons champagne vinegar
- ¼ cup basil leaves, torn

Directions:
1. In your slow cooker, mix orange juice with sugar, vinegar, oil, blueberries and strawberries, toss to coat, cover, cook on High for 2 hours, divide into bowls, sprinkle basil on top and serve!

Nutrition: Calories 137, Fat 4.2g, Cholesterol 0mg, Sodium 2mg, Carbohydrate 29.3g, Fiber 4.2g, Sugars 18g, Protein 1.8g, Potassium 362mg

Mango and Orange Sauce

Preparation time: 6 hours and 10 minutes | Cooking time: 2 hours | Servings: 3

Ingredients:
- 4 cups mango, peeled and cubed
- 6 tablespoons palm sugar
- 3 tablespoons lime juice
- ¼ cup orange juice

Directions:
1. Put mango, orange juice, lime juice and sugar, stir, cover and cook on High for 2 hours.
2. Divide into bowls and keep in the fridge for 6 hours before serving.

Nutrition: Calories 216, Fat 0.9g, Cholesterol 0mg, Sodium 896mg, Carbohydrate 53.7g, Fiber 3.6g, Sugars 49.3g, Protein 2g, Potassium 1167mg

Sweet Minty Grapefruit Mix

Preparation time: 10 minutes | Cooking time: 2 hours | Servings: 4

Ingredients:
- 1 cup water
- 1 cup palm sugar
- 64 ounces red grapefruit juice
- 2 cups grapefruit, peeled and cubed
- ½ cup mint, chopped

Directions:
1. In your slow cooker, mix the water with your grapefruit, sugar, mint and grapefruit juice, stir, cover and cook on High for 2 hours.
2. Divide into bowls and serve cold.

Nutrition: Calories 554, Fat 0.3g, Cholesterol 0mg, Sodium 3122mg, Carbohydrate 139g, Fiber 2.1g, Sugars 67.4g, Protein 1.3g, Potassium 2775mg

Coconut Banana Cream

Preparation time: 10 minutes | Cooking time: 1 hour | Servings: 4

Ingredients:
- 1 and ½ cup coconut cream
- 2 cups banana, peeled and mashed
- 2 tablespoons maple syrup
- 2 teaspoons lime zest, grated
- 1 tablespoon lime juice

Directions:
1. In your slow cooker, combine the banana with the cream and the other ingredients, put the lid on and cook on High for 1 hour.
2. Divide into bowls and serve cold.

Nutrition: Calories 302, Fat 21.7g, Cholesterol 0mg, Sodium 15mg, Carbohydrate 29.4g, Fiber 4.1g, Sugars 18.3g, Protein 2.9g, Potassium 533mg

Plums Stew

Preparation time: 10 minutes | Cooking time: 2 hours | Servings: 4

Ingredients:
- 16 ripe plums, stoned and halved
- 5 cardamom pods,
- crushed
- 1 cup water
- ½ cup coconut sugar

Directions:
1. In your slow cooker, mix the plums with the water, sugar and cardamom, stir, cover and cook on High for 2 hours.
2. Divide into bowls and serve cold.

Nutrition: Calories 140, Fat 1g, Cholesterol 0mg, Sodium 7mg, Carbohydrate 36.1g, Fiber 4.3g, Sugars 28g, Protein 2.4g, Potassium 445mg

Cinnamon Apples

Preparation time: 10 minutes | Cooking time: 4 hours | Servings: 4

Ingredients:
- A handful raisins
- 4 big apples, cored and cut into wedges
- 2 tablespoons natural
- apple juice
- 2 tablespoons stevia
- 1 tablespoon cinnamon powder

Directions:
1. In your slow cooker, mix the apples with the raisins, cinnamon, apple juice and stevia, cover and cook on Low for 4 hours.
2. Divide into bowls and serve warm.

Nutrition: Calories 151, Fat 1.9g, Cholesterol 0mg, Sodium 17mg, Carbohydrate 40.9g, Fiber 6g, Sugars 25.5g, Protein 1.1g, Potassium 242mg

Figs and Avocado Bowls

Preparation time: 6 minutes | Cooking time: 1 hour | Servings: 2

Ingredients:
- 2 cups avocado, peeled, pitted and cubed
- 1 cup coconut cream
- 1 tablespoon maple
- syrup
- 12 figs, halved
- ½ cup almonds, chopped
- 1 teaspoon vanilla extract

Directions:
1. In your slow cooker, mix the avocado with the cream, maple syrup and the other ingredients, put the lid on, cook on High for 1 hour, divide into bowls and serve.

Nutrition: Calories 1027, Fat 70g, Cholesterol 0mg, Sodium 40mg, Carbohydrate 104.1g, Fiber 26.6g, Sugars 66.6g, Protein 14.3g, Potassium 1997mg

Cocoa Cake

Preparation time: 10 minutes | Cooking time: 2 hours and 30 minutes | Servings: 8

Ingredients:
- 1 cup flour
- 1 and ½ cup stevia
- ½ cup chocolate almond milk
- 2 teaspoons baking powder
- 1 and ½ cups hot water
- ¼ cup cocoa powder+ 2 tablespoons
- 2 tablespoons canola oil
- 1 teaspoon vanilla extract
- Cooking spray

Directions:
1. In a bowl, mix flour with ¼-cup cocoa, baking powder, almond milk, oil and vanilla extract, whisk well and spread on the bottom of the slow cooker greased with cooking spray.
2. In a separate bowl, mix stevia with the water and the rest of the cocoa, whisk well, spread over the batter, cover, and cook your cake on High for 2 hours and 30 minutes.
3. Leave the cake to cool down, slice and serve.

Nutrition: Calories 150, Fat 7.6g, Cholesterol 1mg, Sodium 7mg, Carbohydrate 56.8g, Fiber 1.8g, Sugars 4.4g, Protein 2.9g, Potassium 185mg

Blueberry Pie

Preparation time: 10 minutes | Cooking time: 1 hour | Servings: 6

Ingredients:
- ½ cup whole wheat flour
- Cooking spray
- 1/3 cup almond milk
- ¼ teaspoon baking powder
- ¼ teaspoon stevia
- ¼ cup blueberries
- 1 teaspoon olive oil
- 1 teaspoon vanilla extract
- ½ teaspoon lemon zest, grated

Directions:
1. In a bowl, mix flour with baking powder, stevia, blueberries, milk, oil, lemon zest and vanilla extract, whisk, pour into your slow cooker lined with parchment paper and

greased with the cooking spray, cover and cook on High for 1 hour.
2. Leave the pie to cool down, slice and serve.

Nutrition: Calories 82, Fat 4.2g, Cholesterol 0mg, Sodium 3mg, Carbohydrate 10.1g, Fiber 0.7g, Sugars 1.2g, Protein 1.4g, Potassium 74mg

Coconut Peach Cobbler

Preparation time: 10 minutes | Cooking time: 4 hours | Servings: 4

Ingredients:
- 4 cups peaches, peeled and sliced
- Cooking spray
- ¼ cup coconut sugar
- 1 and ½ cups whole wheat sweet crackers, crushed
- ½ cup almond milk
- ½ teaspoon cinnamon powder
- ¼ cup stevia
- 1 teaspoon vanilla extract
- ¼ teaspoon nutmeg, ground

Directions:
1. In a bowl, mix peaches with sugar, cinnamon, and stir.
2. In a separate bowl, mix crackers with stevia, nutmeg, almond milk and vanilla extract and stir.
3. Spray your slow cooker with cooking spray, spread peaches on the bottom, and add the crackers mix, spread, cover and cook on Low for 4 hours.
4. Divide into bowls and serve.

Nutrition: Calories 249, Fat 11.4g, Cholesterol 0mg, Sodium 179mg, Carbohydrate 42.7g, Fiber 3g, Sugars 15.2g, Protein 3.5g, Potassium 366mg

Cherry and Chocolate Cream

Preparation time: 10 minutes | Cooking time: 1 hour and 30 minutes | Servings: 4

Ingredients:
- 1 cup dark and unsweetened chocolate, chopped
- ½ pound cherries, pitted and halved
- 1 teaspoon vanilla extract
- ½ cup coconut cream
- 3 tablespoons coconut sugar
- 2 teaspoons gelatin

Directions:
1. In the slow cooker, combine the chocolate with the cherries and the other ingredients, toss, put the lid on and cook on Low for 1 hour and 30 minutes.
2. Stir the cream well, divide into bowls and serve.

Nutrition: Calories 526, Fat 39.9g, Cholesterol 0mg, Sodium 57mg, Carbohydrate 47.2g, Fiber 10.8g, Sugars 1.1g, Protein 13.4g, Potassium 141mg

Poached Strawberries

Preparation time: 10 minutes | Cooking time: 3 hours | Servings: 10

Ingredients:
- 4 cups coconut sugar
- 2 tablespoons lemon juice
- 2 pounds strawberries
- 1 cup water
- 1 teaspoon vanilla extract
- 1 teaspoon cinnamon powder

Directions:
1. In your slow cooker, mix strawberries with water, coconut sugar, lemon juice, cinnamon and vanilla, stir, cover, cook on Low for 3 hours, divide into bowls and serve cold.

Nutrition: Calories 69, Fat 0.3g, Cholesterol 0mg, Sodium 18mg, Carbohydrate 14.7g, Fiber 1.8g, Sugars 4.6g, Protein 1g, Potassium 143mg

Poached Bananas

Preparation time: 10 minutes | Cooking time: 2 hours | Servings: 4

Ingredients:
- 4 bananas, peeled and sliced
- Juice of ½ lemon
- 1 tablespoon coconut oil
- 3 tablespoons stevia
- ½ teaspoon cardamom seeds

Directions:
1. Arrange bananas in your slow cooker, add stevia, lemon juice, oil and cardamom, cover, cook on Low for 2 hours, divide everything into bowls and serve with.

Nutrition: Calories 137, Fat 3.9g, Cholesterol 0mg, Sodium 2mg, Carbohydrate 33.5g, Fiber 3.2g, Sugars 14.6g, Protein 1.4g, Potassium 433mg

Orange and Pecans Cake

Preparation time: 10 minutes | Cooking time: 5 hours | Servings: 4

Ingredients:
- Cooking spray
- 1 cup almond flour
- 1 cup orange juice
- 1 cup coconut sugar
- 3 tablespoons coconut oil, melted
- 1 teaspoon baking powder
- ½ teaspoon cinnamon powder
- ½ cup almond milk
- ½ cup pecans, chopped
- ¾ cup water
- ½ cup orange peel, grated

Directions:
1. In a bowl, mix flour with half of the sugar,

baking powder, cinnamon, 2 tablespoons oil, milk and pecans, stir and pour this in your slow cooker greased with cooking spray.
2. Heat up a small pan over medium heat, add water, orange juice, orange peel, the rest of the oil and the rest of the sugar, stir, bring to a boil, pour over the mix in the slow cooker, cover and cook on Low for 5 hours.
3. Divide into bowls and serve cold.

Nutrition: Calories 565, Fat 48.8g, Cholesterol 0mg, Sodium 28mg, Carbohydrate 26g, Fiber 7.8g, Sugars 7.1g, Protein 10.2g, Potassium 459mg

Plums Cake

Preparation time: 10 minutes | Cooking time: 3 hours | Servings: 6

Ingredients:
- 2 cups whole wheat flour
- 1 teaspoon vanilla extract
- 1 and ½ cups plums, peeled and chopped
- ½ cup coconut cream
- 1 teaspoon baking powder
- ¾ cup coconut sugar
- 4 tablespoons avocado oil

Directions:
1. In the slow cooker lined with parchment paper, combine the flour with the plums and the other ingredients and whisk.
2. Put the lid on, cook on High for 3 hours, leave the cake to cool down, slice and serve.

Nutrition: Calories 232, Fat 6.4g, Cholesterol 0mg, Sodium 10mg, Carbohydrate 38.3g, Fiber 2.2g, Sugars 2.7g, Protein 5.1g, Potassium 238mg

Poached Pears

Preparation time: 10 minutes | Cooking time: 4 hours | Servings: 4

Ingredients:
- 2 cups grapefruit juice
- 4 pears, peeled and cored
- ¼ cup maple syrup
- 1 tablespoon ginger, grated
- 2 teaspoons cinnamon powder

Directions:
1. In your slow cooker, mix pears with grapefruit juice, maple syrup, cinnamon and ginger, cover, cook on Low for 4 hours, divide everything into bowls and serve.

Nutrition: Calories 214, Fat 0.5g, Cholesterol 0mg, Sodium 5mg, Carbohydrate 55.3g, Fiber 7.9g, Sugars 40.2g, Protein 1.6g, Potassium 461mg

Pumpkin Pie

Preparation time: 10 minutes | Cooking time: 2 hours | Servings: 10

Ingredients:
- 2 cups almond flour extract
- 1 egg, whisked
- 1 cup pumpkin puree
- 1 and ½ teaspoons baking powder
- Cooking spray
- 1 tablespoon coconut oil, melted
- 1 tablespoon vanilla
- ½ teaspoon baking soda
- 1 and ½ teaspoons cinnamon powder
- ¼ teaspoon ginger, ground
- 1/3 cup maple syrup
- 1 teaspoon lemon juice

Directions:
1. In a bowl, flour with baking powder, baking soda, cinnamon, ginger, egg, oil, vanilla, pumpkin puree, maple syrup and lemon juice, stir and pour in your slow cooker greased with cooking spray and lined with parchment paper, cover the pot and cook on Low for 2 hours and 20 minutes.
2. Leave the pie to cool down, slice and serve.

Nutrition: Calories 91, Fat 4.8g, Cholesterol 16mg, Sodium 74mg, Carbohydrate 10.8g, Fiber 1.3g, Sugars 7.5g, Protein 2g, Potassium 157mg

Carrot Muffins

Preparation time: 10 minutes | Cooking time: 3 hours | Servings: 4

Ingredients:
- 4 tablespoons cashew butter, melted
- 4 eggs, whisked
- ½ cup coconut cream
- 1 cup carrots, peeled and grated
- 4 teaspoons maple syrup
- ¾ cup coconut flour
- ½ teaspoon baking soda

Directions:
1. In a bowl, mix the cashew butter with the eggs, cream and the other ingredients, whisk well and pour into a muffin pan that fits the slow cooker.
2. Put the lid on, cook the muffins on High for 3 hours, cool down and serve.

Nutrition: Calories 345, Fat 21.7g, Cholesterol 164mg, Sodium 247mg, Carbohydrate 28.6g, Fiber 10.7g, Sugars 6.7g, Protein 12.3g, Potassium 327mg

Lemon Cream

Preparation time: 10 minutes | Cooking time: 3 hours | Servings: 10

Ingredients:
- 2 pounds lemons, washed, peeled and sliced

- 2 pounds coconut sugar
- 1 tablespoon vinegar

Directions:
1. In your slow cooker, mix lemons with coconut sugar and vinegar, stir, cover, cook on High for 3 hours, blend using an immersion blender, divide into small bowls and serve.

Nutrition: Calories 46, Fat 0.3g, Cholesterol 0mg, Sodium 10mg, Carbohydrate 12.3g, Fiber 2.5g, Sugars 2.3g, Protein 1.2g, Potassium 126mg

Minty Rhubarb Dip

Preparation time: 10 minutes | Cooking time: 3 hours | Servings: 8

Ingredients:
- 1 cup coconut sugar
- 1/3 cup water
- 4 pounds rhubarb, chopped
- 1 tablespoon mint, chopped

Directions:
1. In your slow cooker, mix water with rhubarb, sugar and mint, stir, cover, cook on High for 3 hours, blend using an immersion blender, divide into cups and serve cold.

Nutrition: Calories 60, Fat 0.5g, Cholesterol 0mg, Sodium 15mg, Carbohydrate 12.7g, Fiber 4.1g, Sugars 2.5g, Protein 2.2g, Potassium 657mg

Cherry Jam

Preparation time: 10 minutes | Cooking time: 3 hours | Servings: 6

Ingredients:
- 2 cups coconut sugar
- 4 cups cherries, pitted
- 2 tablespoons lemon juice
- 3 tablespoons gelatin

Directions:
1. In your slow cooker, mix lemon juice with gelatin, cherries and coconut sugar, stir, cover, cook on High for 3 hours, divide into bowls and serve cold.

Nutrition Calories 171, Fat 0.1g, Cholesterol 0mg, Sodium 41mg, Carbohydrate 37.2g, Fiber 0.7g, Sugars 0.1g, Protein 3.8g, Potassium 122mg

Cinnamon Rice Pudding

Preparation time: 10 minutes | Cooking time: 5 hours | Servings: 4

Ingredients:
- 2 cups white rice
- 1 cup coconut sugar
- 2 cinnamon sticks
- 6 and ½ cups water
- ½ cup coconut, shredded

Directions:
1. In your slow cooker, mix water with the rice, sugar, cinnamon and coconut, stir, cover, cook on High for 5 hours, discard cinnamon, divide pudding into bowls and serve warm.

Nutrition: Calories 400, Fat 4g, Cholesterol 0mg, Sodium 28mg, Carbohydrate 81.2g, Fiber 2.7g, Sugars 0.8g, Protein 7.2g, Potassium 151mg

Orange and Plums Compote

Preparation time: 10 minutes | Cooking time: 2 hours and 30 minutes | Servings: 4

Ingredients:
- ½ pound oranges, peeled and cut into segments
- ½ pound plums, pitted and halved
- 1 cup orange juice
- 3 tablespoons coconut sugar
- ½ cup water

Directions:
1. In the slow cooker, combine the oranges with the plums, orange juice and the other ingredients, put the lid on and cook on High for 2 hours and 30 minutes.
2. Stir, divide into bowls and serve cold.

Nutrition: Calories 130, Fat 0.2g, Cholesterol 0mg, Sodium 31mg, Carbohydrate 28.4g, Fiber 1.6g, Sugars 11.4g, Protein 1.8g, Potassium 240mg

Almond Chocolate Bars

Preparation time: 10 minutes | ooking time: 2 hours and 30 minutes | Servings: 12

Ingredients:
- 1 cup coconut sugar
- ½ cup dark chocolate chips
- 1 egg white
- ¼ cup coconut oil, melted
- ½ teaspoon vanilla extract
- 1 teaspoon baking powder
- 1 and ½ cups almond meal

Directions:
1. In a bowl, mix the oil with sugar, vanilla extract, egg white, baking powder and almond flour and whisk well
2. Fold in chocolate chips and stir gently.
3. Line your slow cooker with parchment paper, grease it, add cookie mix, press on the bottom, cover and cook on low for 2 hours and 30 minutes.
4. Take cookie sheet out of the slow cooker, cut into medium bars and serve.

Nutrition: Calories 141, Fat 11.8g, Cholesterol 0mg, Sodium 7mg, Carbohydrate 7.7g, Fiber 1.5g, Sugars 3.2g, Protein 3.2g, Potassium 134mg

Pineapple Pudding

Preparation time: 10 minutes | Cooking time: 5 hours | Servings: 4

Ingredients:

- 1 cup pineapple juice, natural
- Cooking spray
- 1 teaspoon baking powder
- 1 cup coconut flour
- 3 tablespoons avocado oil
- 3 tablespoons stevia
- ½ cup pineapple, chopped
- ½ cup lemon zest, grated
- ½ cup coconut milk
- ½ cup pecans, chopped

Directions:

1. Spray your slow cooker with cooking spray.
2. In a bowl, mix flour with stevia, baking powder, oil, milk, pecans, pineapple, lemon zest and pineapple juice, stir well, pour into your slow cooker greased with cooking spray, cover and cook on Low for 5 hours.
3. Divide into bowls and serve.

Nutrition: Calories 431, Fat 29.7g, Cholesterol 0mg, Sodium 8mg, Carbohydrate 47.1g, Fiber 17g, Sugars 10.9g, Protein 8.1g, Potassium 482mg

Delicious Apple Mix

Preparation time: 10 minutes | Cooking time: 4 hours | Servings: 4

Ingredients:

- 6 big apples, roughly chopped
- Cooking spray
- ½ cup almond flour
- ½ cup walnuts, chopped
- ¼ cup coconut oil, melted
- 2 teaspoons lemon juice
- 3 tablespoons stevia
- ¼ teaspoon ginger, grated
- ¼ teaspoon cinnamon powder

Directions:

1. Spray your slow cooker with cooking spray.
2. In a bowl, mix stevia with lemon juice, ginger, apples and cinnamon, stir and pour into your slow cooker.
3. In another bowl, mix flour with walnuts and oil, stir, pour into the slow cooker, cover, and cook on Low for 4 hours.
4. Divide into bowls and serve.

Nutrition: Calories 474, Fat 30.3g, Cholesterol 0mg, Sodium 9mg, Carbohydrate 58.4g, Fiber 10.7g, Sugars 35g, Protein 7.7g, Potassium 444mg

Grapes Compote

Preparation time: 10 minutes | Cooking time: 2 hours | Servings: 4

Ingredients:

- 4 tablespoons coconut sugar
- 1 and ½ cups water
- 1 pound green grapes
- 1 teaspoon vanilla extract

Directions:

1. In your slow cooker, combine the grapes with the sugar and the other ingredients, put the lid on and cook on High for 2 hours, divide into bowls and serve.

Nutrition: Calories 227, Fat 1.5g, Cholesterol 0mg, Sodium 45mg, Carbohydrate 47.6g, Fiber 2.3g, Sugars 18.8g, Protein 3.6g, Potassium 271mg

Avocado Pudding

Preparation time: 6 minutes | Cooking time: 1 hour | Servings: 4

Ingredients:

- ½ cup coconut water
- 2 teaspoons lime zest, grated
- 2 tablespoons green tea powder
- 1 and ½ cup avocado, pitted, peeled and chopped
- 1 tablespoon stevia

Directions:

1. In your slow cooker, mix coconut water with avocado, green tea powder, lime zest and stevia, stir, cover, cook on Low for 1 hour, divide into bowls and serve.

Nutrition: Calories 120, Fat 10.7g, Cholesterol 0mg, Sodium 35mg, Carbohydrate 8.5g, Fiber 4.4g, Sugars 1.1g, Protein 1.5g, Potassium 362mg

Chia Pudding

Preparation time: 10 minutes | Cooking time: 1 hour | Servings: 4

Ingredients:

- ½ cup pumpkin puree
- 2 tablespoons maple syrup
- 1 and ½ cup coconut milk
- ½ cup chia seeds
- ¼ teaspoon ginger, grated
- ½ teaspoon cinnamon powder

Directions:

1. In your slow cooker, mix the milk with the pumpkin puree, maple syrup, chia, cinnamon and ginger, stir, cover, cook on High for 1 hour, divide into bowls and serve.

Nutrition: Calories 366, Fat 29.3g, Cholesterol 0mg, Sodium 20mg, Carbohydrate 24.8g, Fiber 11.5g, Sugars 10g, Protein 6.6g, Potassium 423mg

Grapefruit Compote

Preparation time: 10 minutes | Cooking time: 2 hours | Servings: 6

Ingredients:
- 64 ounces red grapefruit juice
- 1 cup honey
- ½ cup mint, chopped
- 1 cup water
- 2 grapefruits, peeled and chopped

Directions:
1. In your slow cooker, mix grapefruit with water, honey, mint and grapefruit juice, stir, cover, cook on High for 2 hours, divide into bowls and serve cold.

Nutrition: Calories 364, Fat 0.1g, Cholesterol 0mg, Sodium 52mg, Carbohydrate 94.9g, Fiber 1.1g, Sugars 49.4g, Protein 0.7g, Potassium 124mg

Dark Cherry and Cocoa Compote

Preparation time: 10 minutes | Cooking time: 2 hours | Servings: 6

Ingredients:
- 1 pound dark cherries, pitted and halved
- ¾ cup red grape juice
- ¼ cup maple syrup
- ½ cup dark cocoa powder
- 2 tablespoons stevia
- 2 cups water

Directions:
1. In your slow cooker, mix cocoa powder with grape juice, maple syrup, cherries, water and stevia, stir, cover, cook on High for 2 hours, divide into bowls and serve cold.

Nutrition: Calories 132, Fat 1.4g, Cholesterol 0mg, Sodium 179mg, Carbohydrate 37.9g, Fiber 7g, Sugars 23g, Protein 3.2g, Potassium 28mg

Creamy Grapes Bowls

Preparation time: 10 minutes | Cooking time: 2 hours | Servings: 4

Ingredients:
- 1 pound green grapes
- 3 tablespoons coconut sugar
- 1 and ½ cups coconut cream
- 2 teaspoons vanilla extract

Directions:
1. In the slow cooker, combine the grapes with the cream and the other ingredients, put the lid on and cook on High for 2 hours.
2. Divide into bowls and serve.

Nutrition: Calories 360, Fat 21.9g, Cholesterol 0mg, Sodium 46mg, Carbohydrate 39g, Fiber 3g, Sugars 21.7g, Protein 3.5g, Potassium 456mg

Citrus Apples and Pears Mix

Preparation time: 10 minutes | Cooking time: 1 hour | Servings: 6

Ingredients:
- 1 quart water
- 5 star anise
- 2 tablespoons stevia
- ½ pound pears, cored and cut into wedges
- ½ pound apple, cored and cut into wedges
- Zest of 1 orange, grated
- Zest of 1 lemon, grated
- 2 cinnamon sticks

Directions:
1. Put the water, stevia, apples, pears, star anise, and cinnamon, orange and lemon zest in your slow cooker, cover, cook on High for 1 hour, divide into bowls and serve cold.

Nutrition: Calories 43, Fat 0.4g, Cholesterol 0mg, Sodium 6mg, Carbohydrate 14.3g, Fiber 2.7g, Sugars 5.9g, Protein 0.7g, Potassium 109mg

Pears Cake

Preparation time: 10 minutes | Cooking time: 2 hours and 30 minutes | Servings: 6

Ingredients:
- 3 cups pears, cored and cubed
- 2 cups coconut flour
- 3 tablespoons stevia
- 2 eggs
- 1 tablespoon vanilla extract
- 1 tablespoon pumpkin pie spice
- 1 tablespoon baking powder
- 1 tablespoon avocado oil

Directions:
1. In a bowl mix eggs with the oil, spice, vanilla, pears and stevia and whisk well
2. In another bowl, mix baking powder with flour, stir, add to apples mix, stir again, transfer to your slow cooker, cover, cook on High for 2 hours and 30 minutes, slice and serve cold.

Nutrition: Calories 22, Fat 6g, Cholesterol 55mg, Sodium 25mg, Carbohydrate 46.2g, Fiber 18.8g, Sugars 8.3g, Protein 7.6g, Potassium 382mg

Walnuts and Avocado Bowls

Preparation time: 10 minutes | Cooking time: 1 hour | Servings: 2

Ingredients:
- 2 cups avocado, peeled, pitted and cubed
- 1 cup walnuts, chopped
- 1 tablespoon lime zest, grated
- 1 tablespoon lime juice
- 1 tablespoon coconut sugar
- ½ cup dark chocolate chips
- ½ teaspoon vanilla

extract
- 1 and ½ cups coconut cream

Directions:
1. In the slow cooker, combine the avocado with the walnuts, lime zest and the other ingredients, put the lid on and cook on High for 1 hour
2. Divide into bowls and serve.

Nutrition: Calories 646, Fat 58.1g, Cholesterol 0mg, Sodium 29mg, Carbohydrate 29.6g, Fiber 9.2g, Sugars 11.9g, Protein 12.3g, Potassium 760mg

Cocoa Pudding

Preparation time: 10 minutes | Cooking time: 1 hour | Servings: 2

Ingredients:
- 2 cups coconut milk, hot
- 2 tablespoons water
- 4 tablespoons cocoa powder
- 4 tablespoons stevia
- 2 tablespoon gelatin

Directions:
1. In a bowl, mix milk with stevia and cocoa powder and stir well.
2. Add the gelatin mixed with water, stir well, add to your slow cooker, cook on High for 1 hour, divide into bowls and serve cold.

Nutrition: Calories 599, Fat 58.6g, Cholesterol 0mg, Sodium 52mg, Carbohydrate 39.2g, Fiber 8.5g, Sugars 8.2g, Protein 13.4g, Potassium 903mg

Raspberry Energy Bars

Preparation time: 10 minutes | Cooking time: 1 hour | Servings: 12

Ingredients:
- 1 cup raspberries
- ½ cup low-fat butter
- ½ cup coconut, unsweetened and shredded
- ½ cup coconut oil, melted
- 3 tablespoons stevia

Directions:
1. In your slow cooker, mix the butter with the oil, coconut, raspberries and stevia, toss, cover and cook on High for 1 hour.
2. Spread on a lined baking sheet, keep in the fridge for a few hours, cut into bars and serve.

Nutrition: Calories 112, Fat 10.4g, Cholesterol 0mg, Sodium 37mg, Carbohydrate 7.7g, Fiber 8.5g, Sugars 8.2g, Protein 13.4g, Potassium 903mg

Berries Cream

Preparation time: 10 minutes | Cooking time: 1 hour | Servings: 10

Ingredients:
- 8 ounces mascarpone cheese
- 1 cup coconut cream
- 1 teaspoon stevia
- 1 pint blueberries

Directions:
1. In your slow cooker, mix the cream with stevia, mascarpone and the blueberries, stir, cover, cook on Low for 1 hour, divide bowls and serve cold.

Nutrition: Calories 118, Fat 8.8g, Cholesterol 12mg, Sodium 23mg, Carbohydrate 8.4g, Fiber 1.5g, Sugars 4.9g, Protein 3.4g, Potassium 118mg

Apple and Rice Bowls

Preparation time: 10 minutes | Cooking time: 2 hours and 30 minutes | Servings: 4

Ingredients:
- 1 cup green apples, cored and cubed
- 1 and ½ cups white rice
- 2 and ½ cups coconut milk
- 2 tablespoons maple syrup
- 1 tablespoons apple pie spice
- 1 tablespoon vanilla extract

Directions:
1. In the slow cooker, combine the apples with the rice and the other ingredients, put the lid on and cook on High for 2 hours and 30 minutes.
2. Divide everything into bowls and serve.

Nutrition: Calories 667, Fat 36.5g, Cholesterol 0mg, Sodium 28mg, Carbohydrate 79.6g, Fiber 5.8g, Sugars 17.4g, Protein 8.6g, Potassium 568mg

Blackberries and Cocoa Pudding

Preparation time: 10 minutes | Cooking time: 1 hour | Servings: 4

Ingredients:
- 3 tablespoons cocoa powder
- 2 cups blackberries
- 14 ounces coconut cream
- 2 tablespoons stevia

Directions:
1. In your slow cooker, mix the cream with cocoa, stevia and blackberries, stir, cover, cook on High for 1 hour, divide into dessert cups and serve cold.

Nutrition: Calories 268, Fat 24.5g, Cholesterol 0mg, Sodium 16mg, Carbohydrate 19.6g, Fiber 7.2g, Sugars 6.9g, Protein 4g, Potassium 479mg

Peach Compote

Preparation time: 10 minutes | Cooking time: 1

hour and 30 minutes | Servings: 6

Ingredients:
- 4 cups peaches, cored and roughly chopped
- 4 tablespoons palm sugar
- 2 teaspoons lemon zest, grated
- 6 tablespoons natural apple juice

Directions:
1. In your slow cooker, mix peaches with sugar, apple juice and lemon zest, stir, cover, cook on High for 1 hour and 30 minutes, divide into bowls and serve cold.

Nutrition: Calories 71, Fat 0.3g, Cholesterol 0mg, Sodium 325mg, Carbohydrate 17.3g, Fiber 1.7g, Sugars 16.7g, Protein 1g, Potassium 473mg

Zucchini Cake

Preparation time: 10 minutes | Cooking time: 4 hours | Servings: 6

Ingredients:
- 1 cup natural applesauce
- 2 cups zucchini, grated
- 3 eggs, whisked
- 1 tablespoon vanilla extract
- 4 tablespoons stevia
- Cooking spray
- 2 and ½ cups coconut flour
- ½ cup baking cocoa powder
- 1 teaspoon cinnamon powder
- 1 teaspoon baking soda
- ¼ teaspoon baking powder

Directions:
1. Grease your slow with cooking spray, add zucchini, sugar, vanilla, eggs, applesauce, flour, cocoa powder, baking soda, baking powder and cinnamon, whisk, cook on High for 4 hours, cool down, slice and serve.

Nutrition: Calories 286, Fat 10.1g, Cholesterol 82mg, Sodium 350mg, Carbohydrate 42.5g, Fiber 18.7g, Sugars 7.9g, Protein 11g, Potassium 153mg

Maple Apple Bowls

Preparation time: 10 minutes | Cooking time: 2 hours | Servings: 4

Ingredients:
- 1 pound green apples, cored and cut into wedges
- ½ cups coconut cream
- 1 teaspoon cinnamon powder
- 2 tablespoons walnuts, chopped
- 1 tablespoon maple syrup

Directions:
1. In the slow cooker, combine the apples with the cream and the other ingredients, toss, put the lid on and cook on High for 2 hours.

2. Divide into bowls and serve warm.

Nutrition: Calories 135, Fat 9.6g, Cholesterol 0mg, Sodium 6mg, Carbohydrate 13.1g, Fiber 2.3g, Sugars 9.8g, Protein 1.8g, Potassium 169mg

Grapes Pudding

Preparation time: 5 minutes | Cooking time: 1 hour | Servings: 4

Ingredients:
- 2 cups coconut milk
- 2 cups grapes, halved
- 1 cup coconut flakes
- 3 tablespoons stevia
- 1 tablespoon coconut oil
- ½ teaspoon cinnamon powder
- ½ cup walnuts, chopped

Directions:
1. In your slow cooker, combine the milk with stevia, oil, coconut, cinnamon, grapes and walnuts, stir, cover, cook on High for 1 hour, divide into bowls and serve cold.

Nutrition: Calories 504, Fat 48.1g, Cholesterol 0mg, Sodium 23mg, Carbohydrate 26.6g, Fiber 5.9g, Sugars 12.9g, Protein 7.5g, Potassium 556mg

Apricot Cream

Preparation time: 10 minutes | Cooking time: 3 hours | Servings: 10

Ingredients:
- 2 pounds apricots, chopped
- 2 tablespoons lemon juice
- 4 cups coconut sugar
- 1 teaspoon cinnamon powder
- 1 teaspoon vanilla extract

Directions:
1. In your slow cooker, mix the apricots with the sugar, lemon juice, cinnamon and vanilla, cover, cook on Low for 3 hours, blend using an immersion blender, divide into bowls and serve cold.

Nutrition: Calories 83, Fat 0.6g, Cholesterol 0mg, Sodium 18mg, Carbohydrate 17.7g, Fiber 1.8g, Sugars 8.3g, Protein 1.6g, Potassium 239mg

Poached Apples

Preparation time: 10 minutes | Cooking time: 4 hours | Servings: 6

Ingredients:
- 6 apples, cored, peeled and sliced
- 1 cup coconut sugar
- 1 cup apple juice, natural
- 1 tablespoon cinnamon powder
- Cooking spray

Directions:

1. Grease your slow cooker with cooking spray, add apples, juice, sugar and cinnamon, stir, cover, cook on High for 4 hours, divide into bowls and serve cold.

Nutrition: Calories 151, Fat 0.5g, Cholesterol 0mg, Sodium 10mg, Carbohydrate 38.6g, Fiber 5.5g, Sugars 27.2g, Protein 0.8g, Potassium 280mg

Lemon Cream

Preparation time: 10 minutes | Cooking time: 1 hour | Servings: 4

Ingredients:
- Juice of 2 lemons
- Zest of 2 lemons, grated
- 1 cup low-fat cream cheese
- ½ teaspoon vanilla extract
- 2 tablespoons coconut sugar
- 1 and ½ cups coconut cream

Directions:
1. In the slow cooker, combine the cream cheese with the lemon juice, zest and the other ingredients, put the lid on and cook on High for 1 hour.
2. Divide the cream into bowls and serve cold.

Nutrition: Calories 324, Fat 22.4g, Cholesterol 5mg, Sodium 350mg, Carbohydrate 21.8g, Fiber 3.2g, Sugars 4.4g, Protein 11.4g, Potassium 390mg

Stewed Cardamom Pears

Preparation time: 10 minutes | Cooking time: 4 hours | Servings: 4

Ingredients:
- 5 cardamom pods
- 2 cups apple juice
- 4 pears, peeled and tops cut off and cored
- 1-inch ginger, grated
- ¼ cup maple syrup

Directions:
1. Put the pears in your slow cooker, add cardamom, apple juice, maple syrup and ginger, cover, cook on Low for 4 hours, divide into bowls and serve.

Nutrition: Calories 241, Fat 0.7g, Cholesterol 0mg, Sodium 10mg, Carbohydrate 61.7g, Fiber 7.6g, Sugars 44.2g, Protein 1.2g, Potassium 454mg

Maple Grapes Compote

Preparation time: 10 minutes | Cooking time: 4 hours | Servings: 2

Ingredients:
- 12 ounces red grape juice
- 1 cup maple syrup
- 2 cups green grapes, halved
- 1 cup water

Directions:
1. In your slow cooker, mix grapes with water, maple syrup and grape juice, stir, cover, cook on Low for 4 hours, divide into bowls and serve cold.

Nutrition: Calories 593, Fat 0.6g, Cholesterol 0mg, Sodium 34mg, Carbohydrate 152.6g, Fiber 0.8g, Sugars 138.5g, Protein 0.6g, Potassium 498mg

Brown Rice Pudding

Preparation time: 10 minutes | Cooking time: 4 hours | Servings: 6

Ingredients:
- 14 ounces low-fat coconut milk
- 2/3 cup brown rice
- 1 and 2/3 cups low-fat milk
- 1 teaspoon vanilla extract
- ½ cup raisins
- 2 tablespoons stevia
- 1 teaspoon cinnamon powder

Directions:
1. In your slow cooker, mix the coconut milk with the low-fat milk, stevia, vanilla, cinnamon and raisins and whisk well.
2. Add the rice, stir, cover and cook on Low for 4 hours.
3. Divide into bowls and serve warm.

Nutrition: Calories 295, Fat 17.1g, Cholesterol 3mg, Sodium 42mg, Carbohydrate 36.1g, Fiber 2.6g, Sugars 13g, Protein 5.7g, Potassium 424mg

Berries Compote

Preparation time: 10 minutes | Cooking time: 2 hours | Servings: 4

Ingredients:
- 1 cup water
- 1 cup blackberries
- 1 cup strawberries, halved
- 1 cup blueberries
- ¼ cup coconut sugar
- Juice of 1 lime
- 2 teaspoons vanilla extract

Directions:
1. In your slow cooker, mix the berries with the water, sugar and the other ingredients, put the lid on and cook on Low for 2 hours.
2. Divide into bowls and serve cold.

Nutrition: Calories 62, Fat 0.4g, Cholesterol 0mg, Sodium 6mg, Carbohydrate 13.9g, Fiber 3.6g, Sugars 7.6g, Protein 1.1g, Potassium 158mg

Berry Cobbler

Preparation time: 10 minutes | Cooking time: 2 hours and 30 minutes | Servings: 8

Ingredients:

- 1 and ¼ cups almond flour
- 1 cup coconut sugar
- 2 cups raspberries
- 2 cups blueberries
- 1 egg
- Cooking spray
- ¼ cup low-fat milk
- 1 teaspoon baking powder
- ½ teaspoon cinnamon powder
- 2 tablespoons olive oil

Directions:

1. In a bowl, mix the almond flour with the sugar, baking powder and cinnamon and stir.
2. In another bowl, mix the egg with the milk, oil, raspberries and blueberries and stir.
3. Combine the 2 mixtures, pour everything into your slow cooker greased with the cooking spray, cover and cook on High for 2 hours and 30 minutes.
4. Divide into bowls and serve.

Nutrition: Calories 196, Fat 12.8g, Cholesterol 21mg, Sodium 23mg, Carbohydrate 15.8g, Fiber 4.8g, Sugars 5.4g, Protein 5.5g, Potassium 157mg

Pumpkin Apple Dip

Preparation time: 10 minutes | Cooking time: 8 hours | Servings: 8

Ingredients:

- 1 cup pumpkin puree
- 8 apples, cored, peeled and sliced
- 1/3 cup water
- 1/3 cup palm sugar
- ½ teaspoon pumpkin pie spice
- ¼ teaspoon nutmeg, ground

Directions:

1. In your slow cooker, combine the apples with the sugar, pumpkin puree, water, spice and nutmeg, stir, cover and cook on Low for 8 hours.
2. Blend using an immersion blender, divide into bowls and serve as a sweet dip.

Nutrition: Calories 167, Fat 0.5g, Cholesterol 0mg, Sodium 491mg, Carbohydrate 43.4g, Fiber 6.3g, Sugars 33.g, Protein 1g, Potassium 713mg

Vanilla Apple, Plums and Grapes Bowls

Preparation time: 10 minutes | Cooking time: 2 hours | Servings: 4

Ingredients:

- 1 pound apples, cored and cut into wedges
- 2 tablespoons coconut sugar
- 1 cup plums, pitted and halved
- 1 cup green grapes
- 1 cup natural apple juice
- 1 teaspoon vanilla extract

Directions:

1. In your slow cooker, combine the apples with the plums, sugar and the other ingredients, put the lid on and cook on Low for 2 hours.
2. Toss, divide into bowls and serve.

Nutrition: Calories 129, Fat 0.2g, Cholesterol 0mg, Sodium 21mg, Carbohydrate 30.3g, Fiber 2.3g, Sugars 17.4g, Protein 0.9g, Potassium 177mg

Apple Dip

Preparation time: 10 minutes | Cooking time: 3 hours | Servings: 4

Ingredients:

- 8 apples, cored and chopped
- 1 teaspoon cinnamon powder
- 2 drops cinnamon oil
- 1 cup water

Directions:

1. Put apples in your slow cooker, add the water, oil and cinnamon, cover, cook on High for 3 hours, blend using an immersion blender, divide into bowls and serve cold.

Nutrition: Calories 297, Fat 7.8g, Cholesterol 0mg, Sodium 6mg, Carbohydrate 61.6g, Fiber 10.8g, Sugars 46.4g, Protein 1.2g, Potassium 478mg

Sweet Pumpkin and Avocado Cream

Preparation time: 10 minutes | Cooking time: 2 hours | Servings: 4

Ingredients:

- 1 cup avocado, peeled, pitted and mashed
- 2 tablespoons coconut sugar
- 1 cup pumpkin puree
- 1 teaspoon vanilla extract
- 1 teaspoon pumpkin pie spice

Directions:

1. In your slow cooker, combine the avocado with the pumpkin purée and the other ingredients, put the lid on and cook on High for 2 hours.
2. Stir, divide into bowls and serve warm.

Nutrition: Calories 147, Fat 7.3g, Cholesterol 0mg, Sodium 26mg, Carbohydrate 18g, Fiber 4.3g, Sugars 2.4g, Protein 1.9g, Potassium 308mg

Cranberry Dip

Preparation time: 10 minutes | Cooking time: 2 hours and 30 minutes | Servings: 4

Ingredients:

- 12 ounces cranberries
- 1 cup coconut sugar
- 2 and ½ teaspoons orange zest, grated
- ¼ cup orange juice
- 2 tablespoons maple syrup

Directions:
1. In your slow cooker, mix orange juice with maple syrup, orange zest, sugar and cranberries, stir, cover and cook on High for 2 hours and 30 minutes.
2. Blend using an immersion blender, divide into bowls and serve.

Nutrition: Calories 35, Fat 0g, Cholesterol 0mg, Sodium 4mg, Carbohydrate 7g, Fiber 1.1g, Sugars 3.4g, Protein 0.1g, Potassium 66mg

Apple Cake

Preparation time: 10 minutes | Cooking time: 3 hours | Servings: 4

Ingredients:
- 1 pound apples, cored and cubed
- 2 teaspoons avocado oil
- 4 eggs, whisked
- 1 cup coconut cream
- 1 cup whole wheat flour
- 1 teaspoon baking powder
- 2 tablespoons coconut sugar

Directions:
1. In a bowl, mix the apples with the eggs and the other ingredients and whisk well.
2. Line the slow cooker with parchment paper, pour the cake mix, put the lid on and cook on High for 3 hours.
3. Slice the cake and serve.

Nutrition: Calories 395, Fat 19.4g, Cholesterol 164mg, Sodium 93mg, Carbohydrate 45.4g, Fiber 3.6g, Sugars 8.2g, Protein 10.8g, Potassium 443mg

Sweet Mango Dip

Preparation time: 10 minutes | Cooking time: 3 hours | Servings: 4

Ingredients:
- 1 tablespoon avocado oil
- 4 mangos, cored and chopped
- 1 apple, cored and chopped
- 2 tablespoons ginger, grated
- ¼ cup raisins
- 1 and ¼ cup coconut sugar
- 1 and ¼ apple cider vinegar
- ½ teaspoon cinnamon
- ¼ teaspoon cardamom powder

Directions:
1. In your slow cooker, mix the oil with cardamom, ginger, cinnamon, mangos, apple, raisins, sugar and cider, stir, cover and cook on High for 3 hours.
2. Blend using an immersion blender, divide into bowls and serve.

Nutrition: Calories 318, Fat 2g, Cholesterol 0mg, Sodium 22mg, Carbohydrate 74.3g, Fiber 7.8g, Sugars 57.5g, Protein 3.8g, Potassium 797mg

Plum Dip

Preparation time: 10 minutes | Cooking time: 3 hours | Servings: 20

Ingredients:
- 2 apples, cored and chopped
- 3 pounds plums, pitted and chopped
- 4 tablespoons cinnamon powder
- 4 tablespoons allspice, ground
- 4 tablespoons ginger, ground
- ¾ pound coconut sugar

Directions:
1. Put plums and apples in your slow cooker, add ginger, cinnamon, allspice and sugar, stir, cover and cook on High for 3 hours.
2. Pulse using an immersion blender, divide into bowls and serve.

Nutrition: Calories 27, Fat 0.2g, Cholesterol 0mg, Sodium 3mg, Carbohydrate 6.6g, Fiber 1.1g, Sugars 3.4g, Protein 0.4g, Potassium 66mg

Plum and Berries Bowls

Preparation time: 10 minutes | Cooking time: 1 hour and 30 minutes | Servings: 4

Ingredients:
- 1 pound plums, stone removed and halved
- 1 cup blueberries
- 1 cup blackberries
- 1 cup coconut cream
- 2 tablespoons coconut sugar

Directions:
1. In your slow cooker, combine the plums with the berries and the other ingredients, put the lid on and cook on High for 1 hour and 30 minutes.
2. Divide into bowls and serve cold.

Nutrition: Calories 229, Fat 14.7g, Cholesterol 0mg, Sodium 30mg, Carbohydrate 23.5g, Fiber 4.3g, Sugars 9.1g, Protein 2.8g, Potassium 270mg

Copyright 2020 by Julia Frazier All rights reserved.

All rights Reserved. No part of this publication or the information in it may be quoted from or reproduced in any form by means such as printing, scanning, photocopying or otherwise without prior written permission of the copyright holder.

Disclaimer and Terms of Use: Effort has been made to ensure that the information in this book is accurate and complete, however, the author and the publisher do not warrant the accuracy of the information, text and graphics contained within the book due to the rapidly changing nature of science, research, known and unknown facts and internet. The Author and the publisher do not hold any responsibility for errors, omissions or contrary interpretation of the subject matter herein. This book is presented solely for motivational and informational purposes only.

Made in the USA
Coppell, TX
20 January 2021